Table of Contents

Keto Slow Cooker Cookbook

Healthy and Easy Low-Carb Keto Diet Recipes for Your CrockPot to Lose Weight Fast

OLIVIA STRATTON

Index

Ketogenic Diet Tips

1. You need to stay hydrated all the time

Specialists recommend drinking 30 oz of water in the first hour once you wake up and add another 30-46 oz of water before noon time. In order to stay properly hydrated you should be drinking at least 100-120 ounces of water on a daily basis.

2. Exercise regularly

Regular resistance training along with running and low-intensity exercise help balance level of sugar in the blood and improve the ability to get into and maintain ketosis.

3. Practice intermittent fasting

If you want to get yourself into ketosis and maintain it, intermittent fasting will be the best option for you, as with intermittent fasting you will reduce calories input and stop consummation of protein or carbs. However, it is strongly recommended to consume low quantities of carbs for at least couple of days before starting intermittent fasting as not to get a hypoglycemic episode.

4. Wisely choose carbs that you consume

Ketogenic diet is a low-carb diet, thus, it is recommended to consume nutrient-rich carbohydrate sources such as non-starchy veggies and small amounts of low-glycemic fruits.

5. Use MCT oil wherever you can

Consumption of high-quality medium chain triglyceride (MCT) oil will allow you to consume more protein/carbs and maintain ketosis. Doing this is probably the best thing you can do to actually get into ketosis and maintain it.

6. Keep stress as low as possible

Stress shuts down the ability to maintain the ketosis. If you are stressing a lot, maybe you should reset your goal to simply stay on a lower carb, anti-inflammatory diet for some time.

7. Get enough sleep

If you do not get enough sleep or the quality of your sleep is poor, you will not be able to get into ketosis and maintain it. Thus, make sure you do get enough sleep.

Slow Cooker Useful Tips

1. Start with carefully reading the instructions for your device

Every slow cooker comes with a manual that you should carefully study, as it contains terms of use, additional useful tips, and, most importantly, information on how use it safely.

2. Try not to open the lid often

Every time you open the lid to check or to stir the dish it adds 15 to 20 minutes of cooking time. Most recipes in this book do not require stirring, so just close the lid and wait till the cooking time is up.

3. Thaw your food

Do not load your slow cooker with icy ingredients (unless it is prepackaged slow cooker meal), as it may create perfect conditions for bacteria to flourish. Thaw vegetables and meat before cooking in your slow cooker.

4. Take care of your slow cooker

If you store the Crockpot insert with food in a refrigerator, let it cool down to the room temperature first. Also, when hot make sure to put the hot insert on a dishtowel first and not straight on a cold counter.

5. Do not overfill your slow cooker

If you cook whole chicken or big roasts, make sure you have a suitable Crockpot size. It is recommended to fill a slow cooker not more than two-thirds full.

6. Brown your food first

If you want to boost your dish flavor, you can just brown the food a bit before transferring it to a slow cooker. This allows you to get an additional caramelized flavor.

7. Store it right

After finishing cooking, wash the cooker and put it into storage. Make sure to check the valves and clean those as well.

Za'atar Chicken

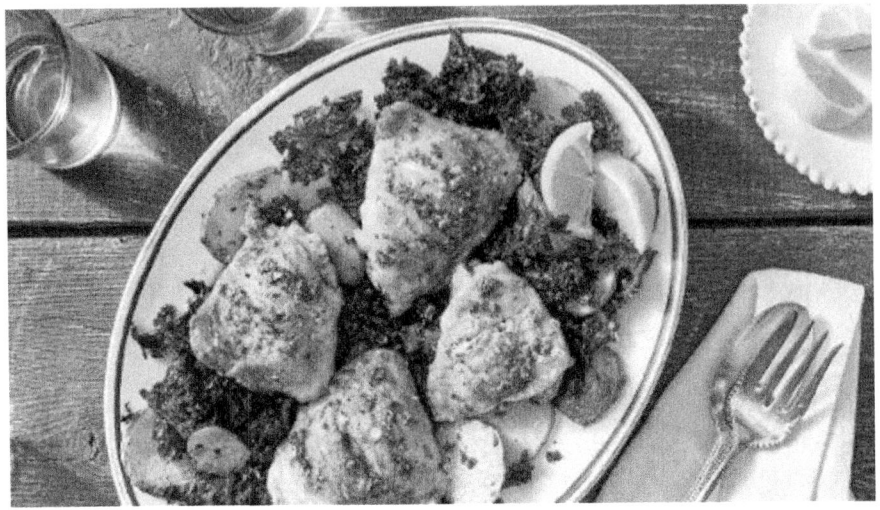

Cooking time: 3-6 hours   **Servings:** 4

Ingredients:

- 3 tablespoons olive oil
- 2 ½ tablespoons lemon zest
- 3 teaspoons garlic, minced
- ¼ cup za'atar herbs
- ½ cup lemon juice
- 1 1/3 teaspoons kosher salt
- 8 chicken 6 to 8 oz thighs, skinless
- 2 lemons, cut in 4 wedges
- 2 green onions bunches, with ends chopped

Instructions:

1. Mix olive oil and za'atar herbs in a bowl, add salt and lemon zest. Add the chicken and coat to cover.

2. Add olive oil to the slow cooker. Put the chicken into slow cooker, add lemons and garlic.

3. Close the lid and cook on Low for 6 hours or on High for 3 hours.

4. Serve topped with green onions.

Nutritional info:

Calories 438; Fats 35g; Net carbs 2.7g; Protein 19.1g

Slow Cooker Chicken Vesuvio

Cooking time: 3-7 hours   **Servings:** 6

Ingredients:

- 1 whole chicken, divided into parts
- 2 tablespoons butter, unsalted
- 1 cauliflower head, cut in florets
- 1 sprig fresh oregano
- 8 garlic cloves
- 1 teaspoon dried thyme
- ¼ cup dry white wine
- ½ cup chicken broth
- 1 teaspoon black pepper
- 1 cup snow peas (optional)
- 2 tablespoons olive oil
- salt, to taste
- parsley

Instructions:

1. Season chicken with salt and pepper.
2. Mix wine, broth, oregano and butter in a bowl.
3. Add olive oil into slow cooker. Put chicken, cauliflower, garlic and peas into the Crockpot, pour wine mixture over it.
4. Close the lid and cook on Low for 7 hours or on High for 3 hours.
5. Serve topped with parsley.

Nutritional info:

Calories 204; Fats 22.3g; Net carbs 5.4g; Protein 16g

Dijon Chicken

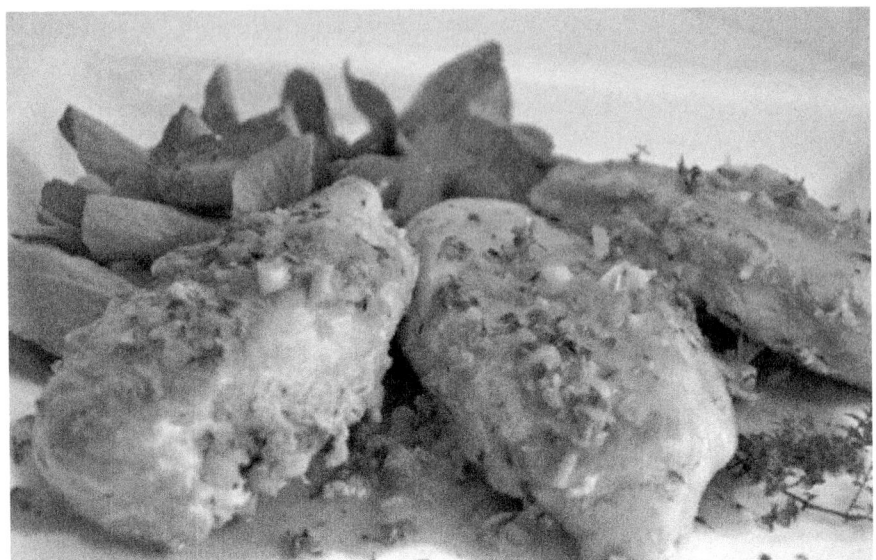

Cooking time: 4-6 hours   **Servings:** 3

Ingredients:

- 3 skinless, boneless chicken breast
- 1 onion, thinly sliced
- 2 garlic cloves, finely chopped
- 1 cup chicken broth
- ½ cup lemon juice

- 1 tablespoon lemon zest
- 3 tablespoons Dijon mustard
- 2 teaspoons dried oregano
- 1 teaspoon salt
- ½ teaspoon ground black pepper

Instructions:

1. Season chicken with salt, pepper and oregano. Put chicken into slow cooker and layer onion over it.

2. Mix broth, mustard, lemon juice and zest in a separate bowl.

3. Pour the mixture over chicken. Cook on Low for 6 hours or for 4 hours on High.

Nutritional info:

Calories 196; Fats 25.6g; Net carbs 7.3g; Protein 18.4g

Chicken Burgers

Cooking time: 3-5 hours   **Servings:** 5

Ingredients:

- 1.5 lb ground chicken
- ½ small onion, minced
- 1 teaspoon dried sage
- 1 egg
- salt and pepper, to taste
- 2 tablespoon butter
- ½ cup water
- almond meal if needed

Instructions:

1. Mix ground chicken, onion, sage, egg, water, salt and pepper in a big bowl. Add almond meal if there is extra liquid in a mixture.

2. Form medium sized patties, about 1 inch thick.

3. Melt butter in a slow cooker, put chicken patties there. Make sure there is enough space between them.

4. Close the lid and cook on Low for 5 hours or on High for 3 hours. The patties should be firm.

5. Serve on buns with vegetables or desired toppings.

Nutritional info:

Calories 315; Fats 25.6g; Net carbs 0.8g; Protein 14.6g

Lemon Marinade Chicken

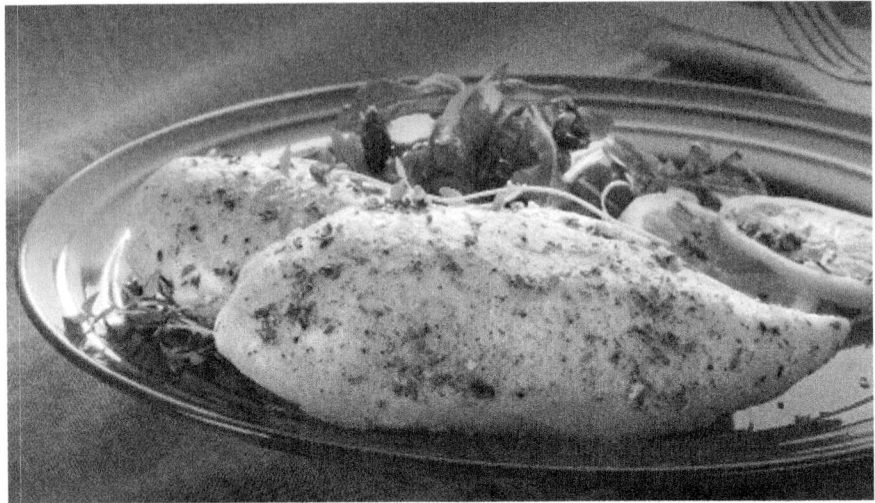

Cooking time: 6-8 hours   **Servings:** 2

Ingredients:

- juice of 1 lemon
- 2 cloves garlic, minced
- 2 tablespoons olive oil
- 1 tablespoon black pepper
- 2 chicken breasts, skinless and boneless
- salt, to taste

Instructions:

1. Mix olive oil, garlic, lemon juice and pepper in a bowl with a fork.
2. Put the chicken breast into the slow cooker and pour the mixture over the chicken.
3. Cook on high with the lid closed for 6 hours or on low for 8 hours.

Nutritional info:

Calories 402; Fats 35.5g; Net carbs 4.1g; Protein 15.7

Chicken & Bean Stew

Cooking time: 4-6 hours

Servings: 4

Ingredients:

- 4 tablespoons olive oil
- 1 big onion, chopped
- 6 strips smoked streaky bacon, chopped
- 8 chicken legs or thighs, skin removed
- 1 tablespoon smoked paprika
- 2 cans diced tomatoes and garlic
- 1 tablespoon dried oregano or mixture of dried herbs
- 2 cans black soy beans
- salt and pepper to taste
- 7 oz water
- cheddar cheese, grated

- low carb tortilla chips

For Low-Carb Sauce:

- 2 oz apple cider vinegar
- 4 oz water
- 2 tablespoons butter
- 1 can tomato paste
- 1 teaspoon onion powder
- 2 teaspoons pepper
- 1 teaspoon Worcestershire sauce
- ½ teaspoon Liquid Smoke Sauce
- salt, to taste

Instructions:

1. Cook the sauce first: mix all the sauce ingredients in a saucepan and bring to a boil over high heat.

2. Turn the heat down to low and simmer for 1 hour while stirring from time to time. Let the sauce cool down and refrigerate.

3. Preheat oil in a slow cooker skillet with the lid closed.

4. Add sliced onions and bacon, cook on High with the lid closed for 1 hour until the onions are soft and slightly browned, the bacon should be crunchy.

5. Put the chicken parts into slow cooker.

6. Add tomatoes, herbs, paprika, sauce, salt, pepper and water.

7. Add beans, close the lid and cook on High for 3-4 hours or on Low for 6 hours, stir occasionally.

8. Check if the chicken is soft. If it is not cover the cooker once again and boil for another 15 minutes.

9. Serve topped with cheddar and tortilla chips.

Nutritional info:

Calories 328; Fats 38g; Net carbs 9.8g; Protein 20g

Chicken Breast & Zucchini Salad

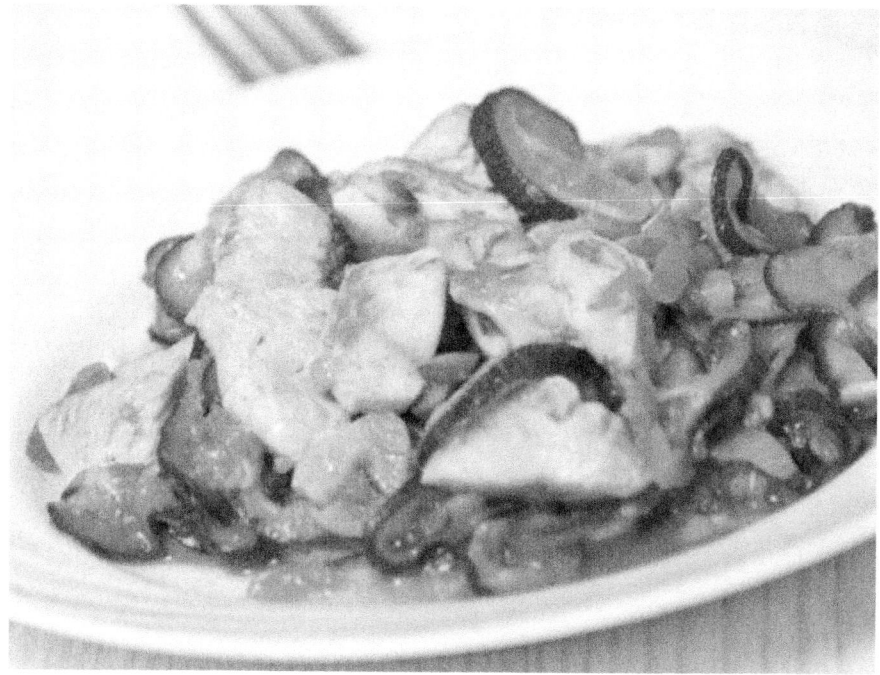

Cooking time: 6 hours   **Servings:** 3

Ingredients:

- ¼ cup olive oil
- 1 lb boneless, skinless chicken breasts
- 11 oz zucchini, thinly sliced
- ¼ cup fresh lemon juice
- ½ red onion, thinly sliced
- coarse salt and ground pepper, to taste
- ¼ cup chopped pecans
- 1 bunch (about 8 oz) spinach, chopped
- ¼ cup Parmesan cheese, grated
- ¼ cup fresh mint, chopped

Instructions:

1. Mix lemon juice, ¼ cup oil, pepper and salt in a bowl.
2. Season zucchini with the mixture.

3. Put some oil to the slow cooker and put chicken into it. Add seasoned zucchini, onion, spinach and mint.

4. Cook on Low for 6 hours.

5. Once cooked add pecans and parmesan cheese.

Nutritional info:

Calories 321; Fats 42.3g; Net carbs 12.1g; Protein 31.3g

Roasted Chicken

Cooking time: 6 hours   **Servings:** 6

Ingredients:

- 1 (4 lb) chicken
- 1 bulb fennel, tops removed, cut into wedges
- 1 yellow onion, thickly sliced
- 1 bunch fresh thyme, plus 20 sprigs
- 1 carrot, cut into 2-inch chunks (optional)
- freshly ground black pepper
- 2 lemons, cut into halves
- 1 head garlic, cut in half crosswise
- 3 tablespoons butter, melted
- 2 tablespoons olive oil
- salt to taste

Instructions:

1. Rinse the chicken and tap dry with a paper towel. Season the chicken with salt and pepper, rub it with garlic and pour butter over it.
2. Stuff the chicken with thyme, garlic, and lemon.
3. Put onions, fennel, and carrots into slow cooker. Season with salt and pepper, add olive oil.
4. Place the chicken on top of vegetables.
5. Close the lid and cook the chicken on Low for 6 hours.
6. Remove the chicken and put it into a baking dish. Preheat the oven to 350 F and cook the chicken in the oven for 4-5 minutes.
7. Slice the chicken and serve with vegetables.

Nutritional info:

Calories 495; Fats 26.1g; Net carbs 8.3g; Protein 16g

Chicken Noodle Soup

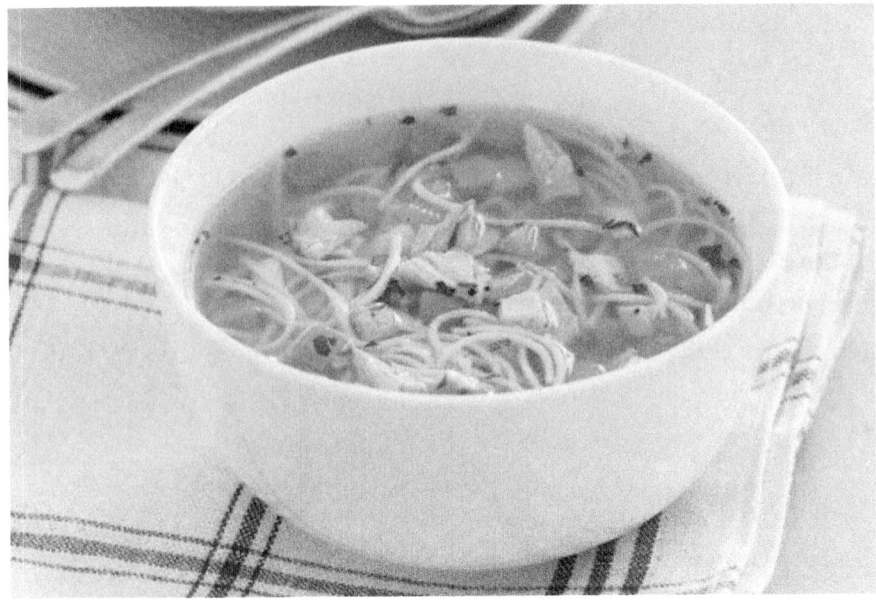

Cooking time: 4-7 hours   **Servings:** 4

Ingredients:

- ½ onion, chopped
- ½ carrot, thinly sliced
- 1 garlic clove, minced
- 8 cups water
- 2 small chicken breasts
- 2 bay leaves
- 1 package cooked Tofu Shirataki noodles, drained and rinsed
- salt, pepper, to taste

Instructions:

1. In a slow cooker mix water, carrot, onion, garlic, bay leaves, salt and pepper.
2. Add chicken breasts to a slow cooker.
3. Close the lid and cook on Low for 6 hours or on High for 3 hours.
4. Once cooked, remove chicken breasts and shred. Remove bay leaves.

5. Add noodles to the slow cooker and cook for 30 minutes on Low with the lid closed.

6. Skim fat from the soup and serve hot.

Nutritional info:

Calories 149; Fats 29g; Net carbs 3.3g; Protein 19.9g

Chicken Salad with Celery and Pecans

Cooking time: 3 hours   **Servings:** 4

Ingredients:

- 2 chicken breasts
- ½ cup water
- ½ onion, diced
- 2 ribs celery, diced
- ½ cup pecans, chopped

For Keto Mayo:

- 1 egg yolk
- ½ teaspoon Dijon mustard
- 2 teaspoons lemon juice
- ½ teaspoon white wine vinegar
- 10 tablespoons avocado oil
- 1/2 teaspoon salt

Instructions:

1. Put chicken, onion, celery and water into a slow cooker. Cook for 3 hours on Low until chicken is cooked.
2. Shred the chicken and drain vegetables. Cool them to room temperature.
3. Meanwhile blend all mayo ingredients in a food processor (for about 30 seconds). The mixture should become lighter and thicker.
4. Slowly add avocado oil to the mixture while blending constantly.
5. Now mix the chicken, vegetables, pecans and mayo in a bowl.
6. Serve separately or with main course.

Nutritional info:

Calories 276; Fats 28.4g; Net carbs 5.6g; Protein 13.6g

Chicken with Thai Peanut Sauce

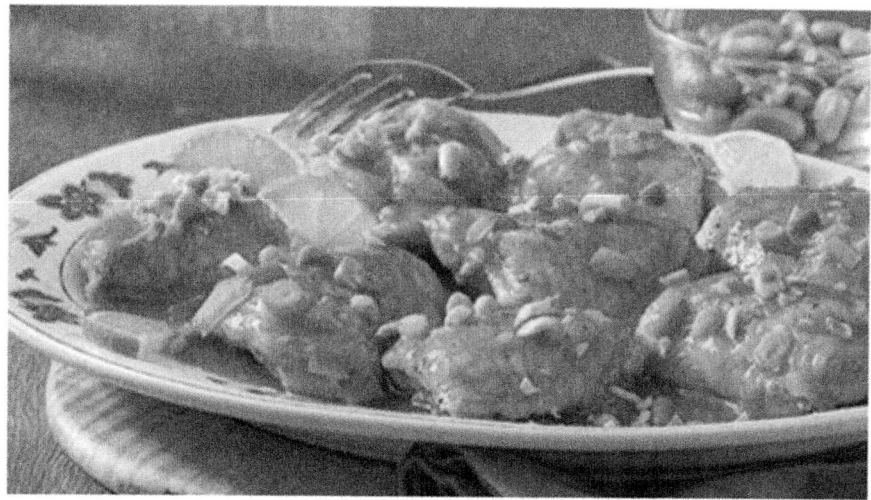

Cooking time: 3-6 hours   **Servings:** 4

Ingredients:

- 4 boneless chicken thighs, cut into bite size pieces
- ½ cup canned coconut milk
- ½ cup unsweetened peanut butter
- 3 tablespoons toasted sesame oil
- 2 tablespoons soy sauce
- 1 tablespoons lime juice
- 1 garlic clove, minced
- 1 teaspoon powdered ginger
- 2 tablespoons peanuts, chopped
- fresh cilantro

Instructions:

1. Put chicken thighs into a slow cooker.

2. Mix coconut milk, peanut butter, garlic, soy sauce and lime juice in a medium bowl.

3. Pour the mixture over chicken. Add some water if the sauce is too thick.

4. Close the lid and cook on Low for 6 hours or on High for 3 hours.

5. You may cut the chicken into pieces and return to the sauce to marinate even better.

6. Serve chicken with spaghetti squash or with salad topped with peanuts and cilantro.

Nutritional info:

Calories 480; Fats 40.6g; Net carbs 6g; Protein 24g

Mexican Chicken Breasts

Cooking time: 4-6 hours   **Servings:** 4

Ingredients:

- 4 chicken breasts, skinless
- 2 tablespoons olive oil
- ½ cup cilantro
- 1 lime, juice
- 1 teaspoon raw honey
- ¼ teaspoon cumin
- 1 yellow onion, chopped
- 3 garlic cloves, minced
- 2 tomatoes, peeled and chopped
- 2 tablespoons parsley, chopped
- 1 teaspoon garlic powder
- 1 tablespoon onion powder
- 1 tablespoon chili powder
- a pinch of sea salt and black pepper

Instructions:

1. Combine chicken, cilantro, onion, garlic cloves, tomatoes and parsley in a bowl.
2. Sprinkle with oil and lime juice and add honey. Season with cumin, garlic powder, onion powder, chili powder, sea salt and black pepper.
3. Transfer to slow cooker and close the lid. *Optional:* you can first brown chicken breasts from both sides in a pan over medium heat.
4. Cook on low for 4-6 hours until chicken is cooked through.

Nutritional info:

Calories 243; Fats 20.4g; Net carbs 7g; Protein 15.7g

Buffalo Chicken Wings

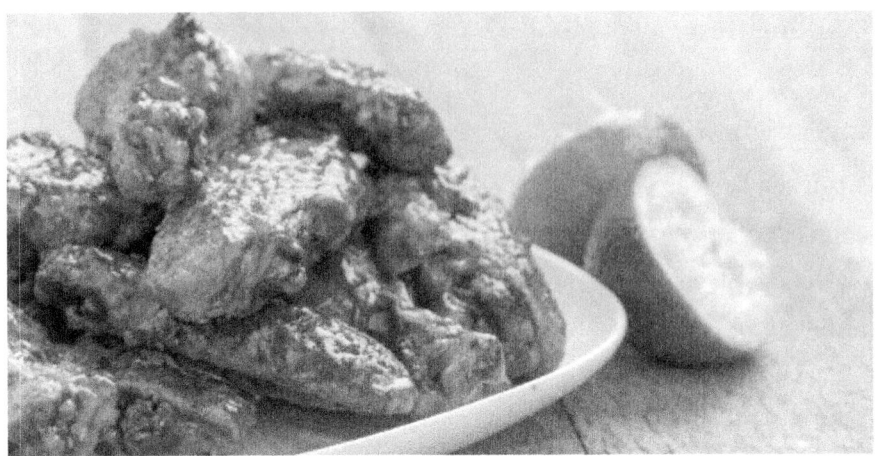

Cooking time: 2-5 hours   **Servings:** 8

Ingredients:

- 3 pounds chicken wings
- ½ cup hot sauce
- 1/3 cup unsalted butter, melted
- ½ teaspoon onion powder
- 2 tablespoons Worcestershire sauce
- salt and pepper, to taste

Instructions:

1. Mix hot sauce, unsalted butter and Worcestershire sauce in the slow cooker.
2. Season chicken wings with salt, pepper and onion powder.
3. Put chicken wings to the slow cooker, stir well to coat with sauce.
4. Close the lid and cook on Low for 4-5 hours or on High for 2 hours.

Nutritional info:

Calories 93; Fats 9.3g; Net carbs 1.4g; Protein 1.4g

Thai Chicken Soup

Cooking time: 6-7 hours   **Servings:** 8

Ingredients:

- 1 ½ pound chicken parts (wings, legs, breast), skinless
- 1 stalk lemongrass, diced
- 10 fresh basil leaves
- 2 tablespoons fresh ginger, sliced
- 1 lime, juiced, for serving
- 2 quarts water (2 liters)
- salt, to taste

Instructions:

1. Put chicken, lemongrass, basil leaves, ginger and water to the slow cooker.
2. Close the lid and cook on Low for 6-7 hours.
3. Remove cooked chicken from the cooker and cut it into bite sized pieces.
4. Return it back to the cooker, close the lid and let cook for 30 minutes on Low.
5. Add lime juice to each plate before serving.

Nutritional info:

Calories 170; Fats 16.4g; Net carbs 2.2g; Protein 14.8g

Chicken Lettuce Wraps

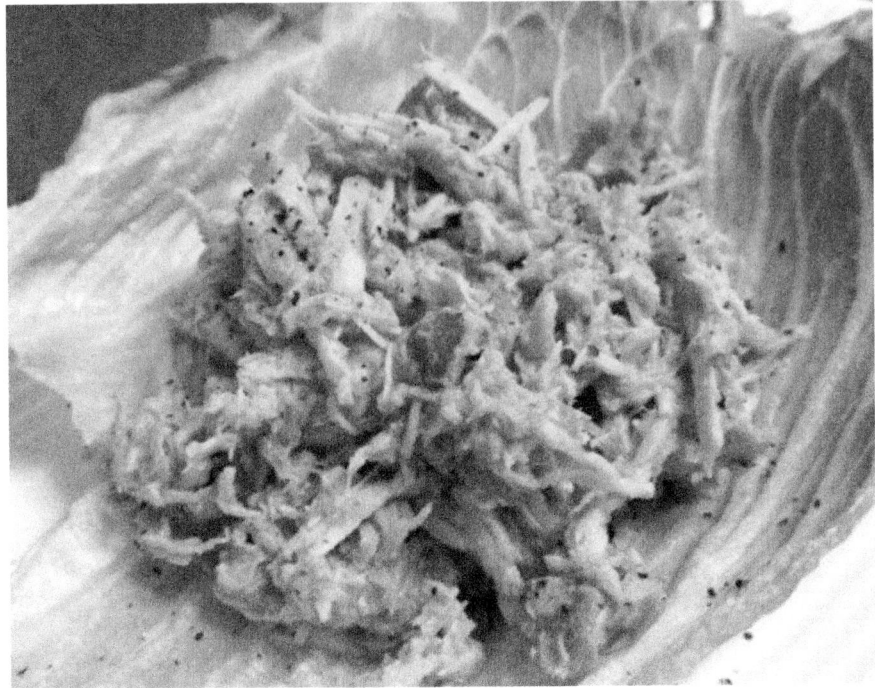

Cooking time: 4.5-8.5 hours   **Servings:** 4

Ingredients:

- 4 chicken breasts, skinless
- 1 onion, chopped
- 2 garlic cloves, minced
- 4 tablespoons hot sauce
- ½ cup low sodium chicken broth
- salt, pepper, to taste
- lettuce leaves, medium

Instructions:

1. Season chicken with salt and pepper. Put breasts into the slow cooker.
2. Add onion, garlic and broth.
3. Close the lid and cook on Low for 4 hours or on High for 8 hours.
4. Open the lid and remove chicken from the cooker.

5. Shred the chicken and return back to the slow cooker, add hot sauce.

6. Close the lid and cook on High for 30 minutes or just keep on warm for 1-2 hours.

7. Serve shredded chicken on lettuce leaves.

Nutritional info:

Calories 137; Fats 11.6g; Net carbs 3.5g; Protein 6.7g

Chicken Cacciatore

Cooking time: 4-8 hours   **Servings:** 5

Ingredients:

- 3 pounds chicken legs with thighs
- 2 garlic cloves, crushed
- 1 teaspoon salt
- 1 teaspoon olive oil
- ½ onion, sliced
- ¼ teaspoon hot pepper flakes
- 2 tablespoons dry red wine
- 1 teaspoon dried oregano
- ½ cup green olives, cut in half
- 1 sprig fresh basil leaves, torn

Instructions:

1. Season chicken with salt, hot pepper flakes and dried oregano. Sprinkle with olive oil.

2. Put the chicken into the slow cooker, add wine, onion, garlic cloves, green olives and fresh basil leaves.

3. Close the lid and cook on Low for 4 hours or on High for 8 hours.

Nutritional info:

Calories 443; Fats 42g; Net carbs 10.6g; Protein 23.1g

Turkey Meatloaf

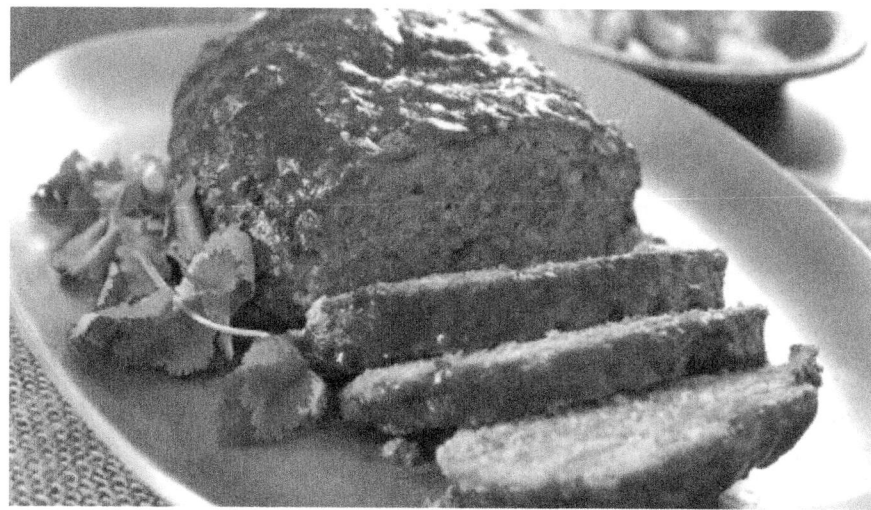

Cooking time: 6-8 hours   **Servings:** 4

Ingredients:

- 2 pounds ground turkey
- ¼ cup almond flour
- 3-4 tablespoons soy sauce
- 1 teaspoon onion powder
- 1 teaspoon garlic cloves, minced
- 1 egg
- salt, pepper, to taste

Instructions:

1. Mix ground turkey with almond flour, soy sauce, onion powder, garlic, egg, salt and pepper.
2. Form into a loaf.
3. Line your Crockpot with a foil. Put the loaf into the slow cooker.
4. Close the lid and cook on Low for 6-8 hours.

Nutritional info:

Calories 478; Fats 26.8g; Net carbs 2.1g; Protein 34.7g

Turkey Meatballs

Cooking time: 6 hours   **Servings:** 6

Ingredients:

- 1 pound ground turkey
- 1 tablespoon olive oil
- 1 onion, sliced
- 1 can diced tomatoes
- ½ cup almond flour
- 1 egg

- 1 teaspoon garlic powder
- 1 teaspoon ginger, ground
- 1 teaspoon dried oregano
- 1 tablespoon soy sauce
- salt, pepper, to taste

Instructions:

1. Mix turkey, almond flour, egg, 1 tablespoon olive oil, garlic powder, ginger, oregano, soy sauce, salt and pepper in a bowl. Form medium sized meatballs.
2. Put sliced onions on the bottom of the slow cooker, add diced tomatoes.
3. Heat oil in a skillet over medium heat. Brown each meatball for 1 minute on each side.
4. Put meatballs on top of onions and tomatoes in the slow cooker.
5. Close the lid and cook on Low for 6 hours.

Nutritional info:

Calories 208; Fats 22.5g; Net carbs 4.2g; Protein 12.8g

Turkey Stew

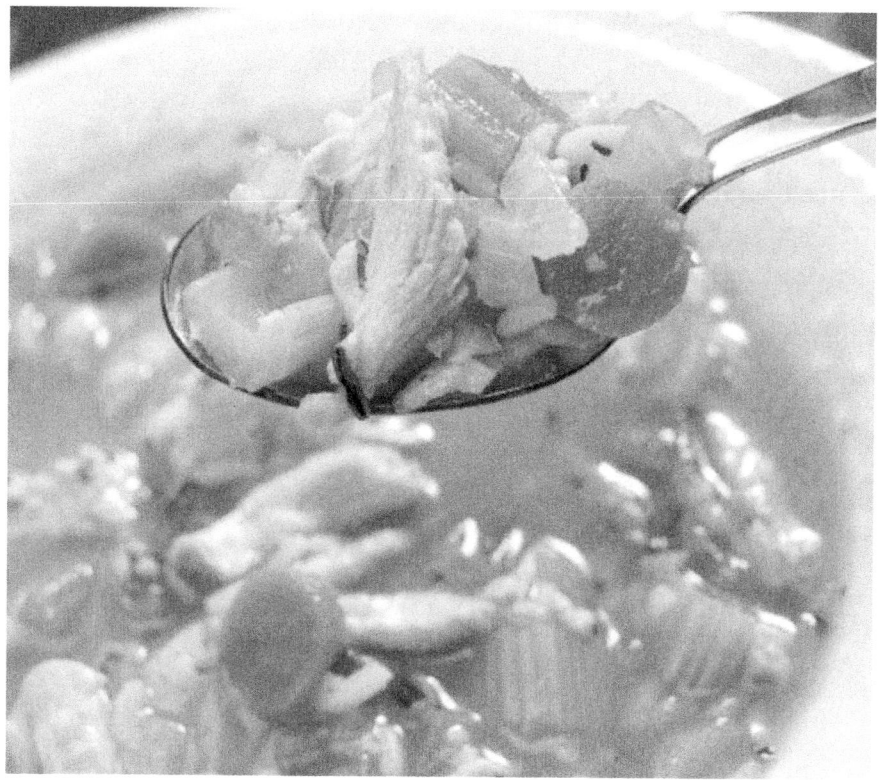

Cooking time: 8 hours   **Servings:** 6

Ingredients:

- 3 cups turkey meat (any part), cooked, cubed
- 1 stalk celery, diced
- ½ onion, diced
- 2 garlic cloves, minced
- ½ cauliflower head florets, diced
- 1 carrot, diced
- 2 cups chicken broth
- 1 teaspoon red pepper flakes
- salt, pepper, to taste

Instructions:

1. Add celery, onion, garlic, cauliflower, carrot and chicken broth to the slow cooker.

2. Season with salt and pepper, add pepper flakes.

3. Close the lid and cook on Low for 8 hours. Add turkey meat 30 minutes before the timer is up and cook till the end.

Nutritional info:

Calories 148; Fats 4.1g; Net carbs 3.9g; Protein 22.9g

Sweet Turkey Tenderloin

Cooking time: 3-4 hours   **Servings:** 6

Ingredients:

- 2 pounds turkey tenderloins
- ½ cup chicken stock
- ¼ cup raw honey
- 2 tablespoons hot sauce
- 1 lime, juiced
- 1 teaspoon ginger, ground
- 1 teaspoon garlic powder
- salt, pepper, to taste

Instructions:

1. Mix chicken stock, raw honey, hot sauce, lime juice, ginger, garlic powder, salt and pepper in a bowl.
2. Put the turkey into the slow cooker and add the chicken stock mixture. Stir well to coat the turkey with the sauce.
3. Close the lid and cook on Low for 3-4 hours.

Nutritional info:

Calories 166; Fats 15g; Net carbs 10.5g; Protein 28.9g

Jalapenos Turkey Chili

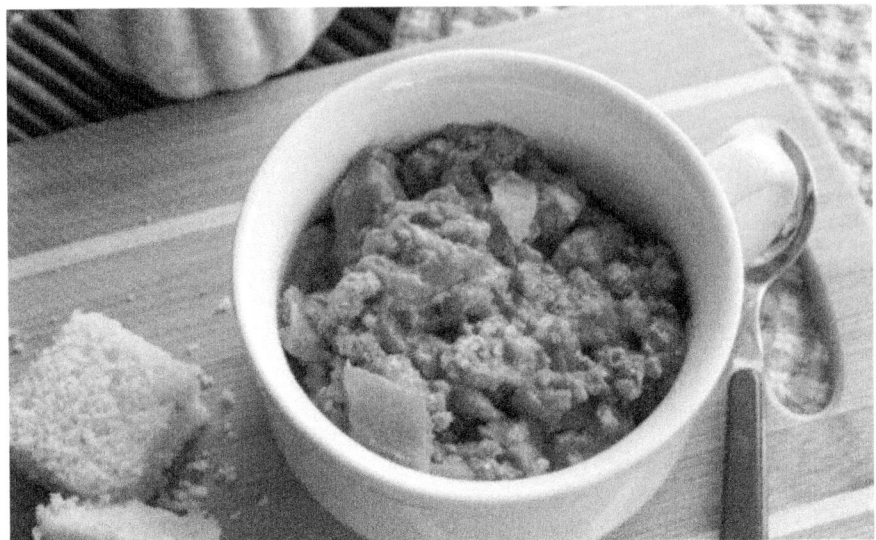

Cooking time: 4-8 hours   **Servings:** 6

Ingredients:

- 1 ½ pound ground turkey
- 1 onion, chopped
- 2 tablespoons olive oil
- 3 garlic cloves, minced
- 2 teaspoons chili powder
- 7 oz (half a can) diced tomatoes
- 2 cups chicken broth
- 2 jalapenos, seeded, chopped
- salt, pepper, to taste

Instructions:

1. Heat oil in a skillet over medium heat. Add ground turkey and cook until slightly brown.

2. Add some oil to the slow cooker or use a cooking spray. Add turkey, onion, garlic, tomatoes, jalapenos and chicken broth.

3. Season with chili powder, salt and pepper.

4. Close the lid and cook on Low for 8 hours or on High for 4 hours.

Nutritional info:

Calories 231; Fats 24g; Net carbs 6.8g; Protein 13.6g

Pumpkin Turkey Chili

Cooking time: 3 hours   **Servings:** 3

Ingredients:

- 1 ½ cups fresh pumpkin, cubed
- 1 can black soy beans
- 1 tablespoon olive oil
- 1 tablespoon chili powder
- 1 ½ tablespoons brown sugar substitute

- 1 onion, chopped
- 2 lb ground turkey
- 1 can (20 oz) diced tomatoes
- 1 tablespoon pumpkin pie spice

Instructions:

1. Preheat olive oil in a pan over low heat for 3 minutes. Add turkey and stir for 7-8 minutes, drain fat.
2. Transfer turkey into the slow cooker and add beans, pumpkin, chili powder, pumpkin pie spice, sugar, diced tomatoes and onion.
3. Cook on High for 3 hours with the lid closed.

Nutritional info:

Calories 300; Fats 42.1g; Net carbs 11.7g; Protein 21.9g

Turkey Breasts

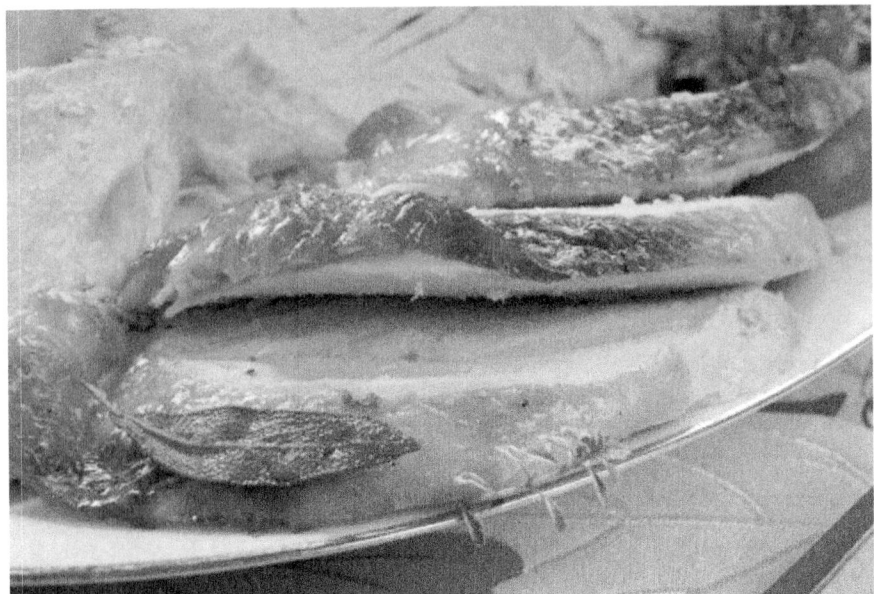

Cooking time: 5-8 hours   **Servings:** 2

Ingredients:

- 4 skinless, boneless turkey breasts
- 2 garlic cloves, minced
- 5 bay leaves

- 2 tablespoons onion powder
- 1 teaspoon dried oregano
- salt and black pepper, to taste
- 2 cups chicken broth

Instructions:

1. Season turkey breasts with salt, pepper, oregano and onion powder. Put the turkey into a slow cooker.

2. Pour broth into a slow cooker; make sure you do not wash off the turkey seasoning. Add garlic and sage leaves.

3. Cook on Low for 8 hours or on High for 1 hour and then on Low for 5 hours.

Nutritional info:

Calories 352; Fats 29.6g; Net carbs 5.9g; Protein 14g

Turkey Cauliflower Rice Soup

Cooking time: 6-7 hours   **Servings:** 4

Ingredients:

- 4 cups chicken or turkey broth
- 1 can tomatoes, diced
- ½ cup carrots, diced
- ½ cup celery, diced
- ½ cup onion, diced
- 2 cups turkey meat, cooked, diced
- ¼ cup cauliflower rice
- salt, pepper, to taste

Instructions:

1. Pour broth into the Crockpot, add tomatoes, carrot, celery and onion, season with salt and pepper.
2. Close the lid and cook on Low for 6-7 hours.
3. Add turkey meat, close the lid and cook on Low for 1 more hour.

Nutritional info:

Calories 112; Fats 12.3g; Net carbs 9g; Protein 14.4g

Turkey Wings

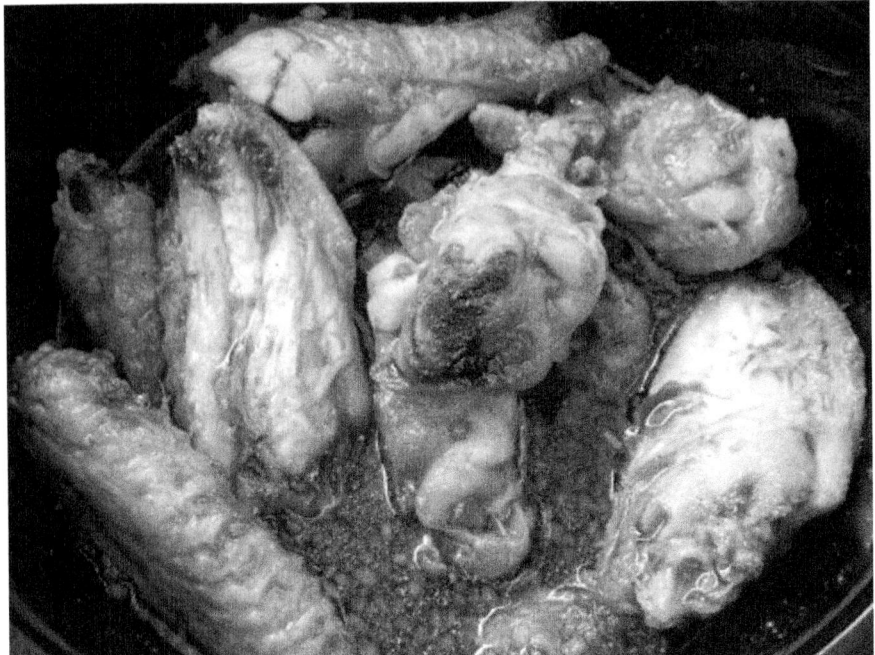

Cooking time: 3-4 hours   **Servings:** 4

Ingredients:

- 6-8 turkey wings
- 1 tablespoon olive oil
- 1 onion, chopped
- ½ cup celery, chopped
- 2 cups chicken or turkey broth
- salt, pepper, to taste

Instructions:

1. Season wings with salt and pepper.
2. Preheat oil in a slow cooker skillet with the lid closed.
3. Add turkey wings and brown them on all sides, for about 5 minutes each side.
4. Remove the wings. Put onion and celery to the Crockpot inner pot, add wings on top.

5. Add broth, close the lid and cook on High for 3-4 hours.

Nutritional info:

Calories 369; Fats 19.7g; Net carbs 3g; Protein 33.7g

Turkey Green Chilies Soup

Cooking time: 6-7 hours   **Servings:** 4

Ingredients:

- 1 lb skinless boneless turkey breast, chopped
- 1 onion, chopped
- 1 garlic glove, minced
- 1 can diced tomatoes with green chilies, undrained
- 2 cups chicken or turkey broth
- 1 tablespoon lime juice
- ¼ teaspoon cayenne pepper
- ½ teaspoon ground ginger
- ½ teaspoon garlic powder
- 1 tablespoon fresh cilantro, minced
- salt, pepper, to taste

Instructions:

1. Mix salt, pepper, cayenne pepper, ground ginger and garlic powder in a bowl. Add turkey meat and toss to coat well.
2. Put turkey to the Crockppot, add onion, garlic, tomatoes, broth, lime juice, add salt and pepper if needed.
3. Close the lid and cook on Low for 6-7 hours.

Nutritional info:

Calories 236; Fats 29.5g; Net carbs 5g; Protein 20.3g

Pulled Turkey

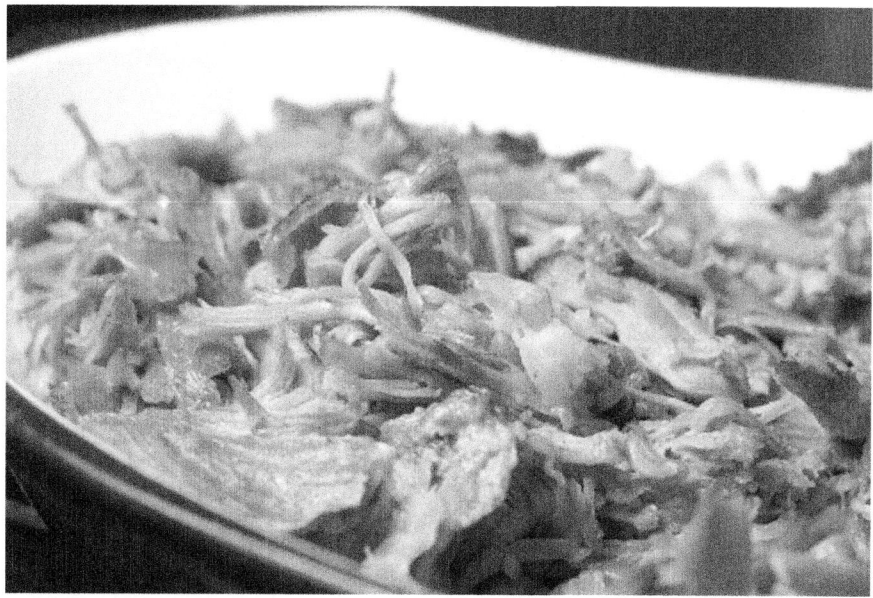

Cooking time: 3-6 hours   **Servings:** 4

Ingredients:

- 4-5 turkey thighs
- 1 onion, chopped
- 1 tablespoon chili powder
- 1 teaspoon ground cumin
- ½ cup reduced sugar ketchup
- 3 teaspoons erythritol or brown sugar Truvia
- 2 tablespoons mustard
- 1 tablespoon apple cider vinegar
- ½ teaspoon salt and ground pepper

Instructions:

1. Put onions into the bottom of the Crockpot.
2. Mix chili powder, cumin, salt and pepper in a bowl, season turkey thighs with the seasoning mixture.
3. Put turkey thighs over the onions.

4. Mix ketchup, mustard and erythritol or brown sugar Truvia and pour over turkey.

5. Close the lid and cook on Low for 5-6 hours or on High for 3-4 hours.

6. Open the lid and let the meat cool for 5-10 minutes. Shred the meat and discard the bones.

7. Add vinegar, salt and pepper to taste.

Nutritional info:

Calories 292; Fats 15.5g; Net carbs 5.8g; Protein 21.5g

Turkey Legs

Cooking time: 6-7 hours   **Servings:** 4

Ingredients:

- 4-6 turkey legs
- 3 teaspoons poultry seasoning
- salt, pepper, to taste
- aluminum foil

Instructions:

1. Wash the turkey legs, season them with salt, pepper and poultry seasoning.
2. Wrap the legs in the foil, each leg in a separate piece.
3. Put the wrapped legs into the Crockpot.
4. Close the lid and cook on Low for 7-8 hours.

Nutritional info:

Calories 241; Fats 10.7g; Net carbs 0.7g; Protein 32g

Beef Filled Lettuce Wraps

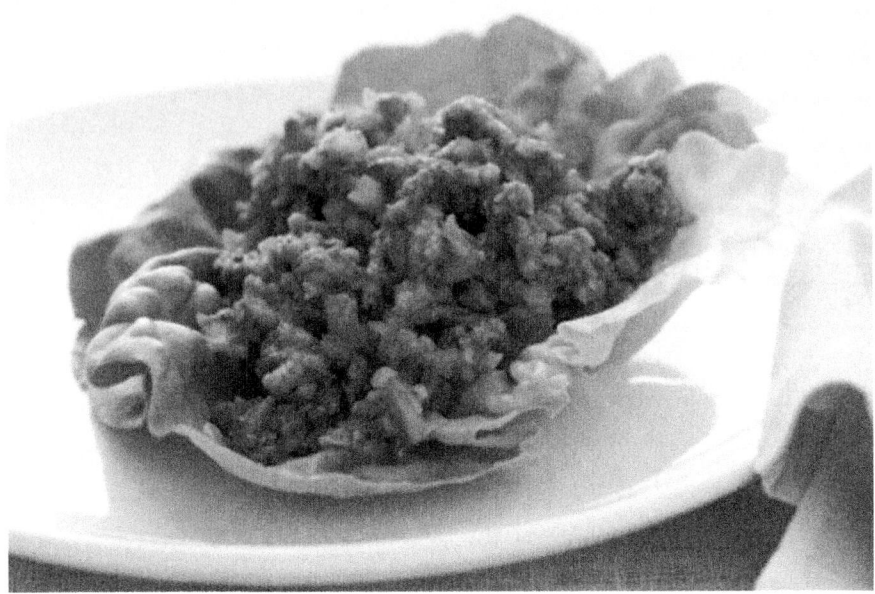

Cooking time: 3 hours 15 minutes   **Servings:** 3

Ingredients:

- 1 lb ground beef
- 2 teaspoons olive oil
- 2 scallions, chopped
- 2 inch piece ginger, grated
- ¼ cup chopped peanuts
- 2 cloves garlic, minced

- 1 head lettuce leaves, separated, cleaned and dried
- 1 teaspoon red pepper flakes
- 1 tablespoon sriracha sauce
- salt and freshly ground black pepper, to taste
- 2 tablespoons soy sauce

Instructions:

1. Preheat oil in a pan and add beef. Cook for 5 minutes stirring and drain the grease.

2. Preheat oil in a slow cooker skillet with the lid closed and then add cooked beef.

3. Add garlic, ginger, soy sauce, scallions, sriracha and red pepper flakes, stir well.

4. Cook on Low for 2-3 hours until brown.

5. Once cooked add peanuts and season with pepper and salt.

6. Serve wrapped in lettuce leaves.

Nutritional info:

Calories 411; Fats 28.9g; Net carbs 8.9g; Protein 20.9g

Meatballs with Spinach

Cooking time: 6 hours   **Servings:** 4

Ingredients:

- 1 lb. ground beef
- 1 (10 oz) package frozen spinach
- ¼ cup parmesan cheese, grated
- 4 cups chicken or beef bone broth
- 1/8 teaspoon ground black pepper
- salt, to taste

Instructions:

1. Mix cheese, salt, pepper, beef, and stir to combine.
2. Roll the mixture into small meatballs.
3. Put meatballs into the slow cooker, add broth, spinach and cook on low for 6 hours.
4. Remove from the heat and sprinkle with additional cheese (optional). Check for seasoning.

Nutritional info:

Calories 484; Fats 38.2g; Net carbs 3.1g; Protein 27.3g

Stir Fried Beef with Veggies

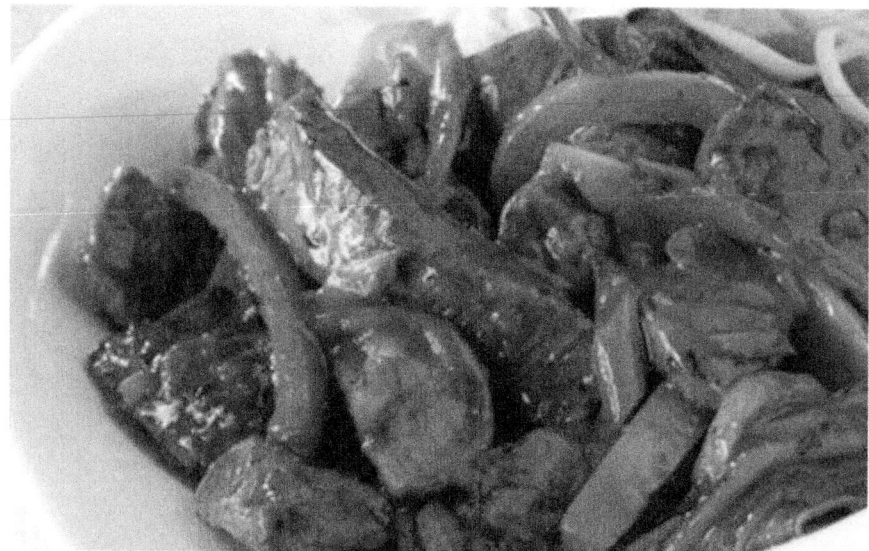

Cooking time: 3-6 hours   **Servings:** 3

Ingredients:

- 1 lb beef sirloin, cut into 1 ½-inch strips
- 2 tablespoons sesame seeds, toasted
- 1½ cups fresh broccoli florets
- 1 carrot, thinly sliced
- 1 onion, chopped
- 2 garlic cloves, minced
- 1 red bell pepper, cut into strips

For Sauce:

- ¼ cup water
- ¼ cup coconut aminos or soy sauce
- 2 tablespoons white vinegar
- 1 teaspoon toasted evoo
- 1 tablespoon ginger
- 1 teaspoon honey

Instructions:

1. Put beef, broccoli florets, carrots, onion, bell pepper and garlic into slow cooker.

2. Mix water, aminos or soy sauce, vinegar, evoo, ginger and honey in a medium bowl.

3. Pour sauce over beef and vegetables.

4. Close the lid and cook on Low for 6 hours or on High for 3 hours.

5. Season with sesame seeds once cooked. Serve with pasta or rice.

Nutritional info:

Calories 477; Fats 31.5g; Net carbs 9.5g; Protein 28.6g

Cheesy Beef Casserole

Cooking time: 3-6 hours   **Servings:** 6

Ingredients:

- 1.5 lbs lean ground beef
- 2 teaspoons olive oil
- 1 tablespoon garlic, minced
- 1 tablespoon tomato paste (can be substituted with tomato puree of 1-2 tomatoes)
- 1 onion, chopped
- 2 cups grated cheddar cheese
- 1 cup low fat cottage cheese
- ¾ cup heavy cream
- 2 cups water
- salt, pepper, to taste

Instructions:

1. Heat oil in a medium pan over high heat. Add ground beef and sauté for 5 minutes. Drain fat and set aside.
2. Clean the pan and heat some more oil in it, add onions and cook for 3 minutes. Add garlic and cook for 30 seconds.
3. Put beef, onion and garlic into a slow cooker. Add water, tomato paste, salt and pepper. Mix well.
4. Close the lid and cook on Low for 6 hours or on High for 3 hours.
5. Open the lid, add cheddar and cottage cheese, heavy cream and stir gently. Close the lid and cook on Low for another 1 hour until the cheese is melted.

Nutritional info:

Calories 473; Fats 27.4g; Net carbs 4.9g; Protein 49.7g

Keto Irish Beef Stew

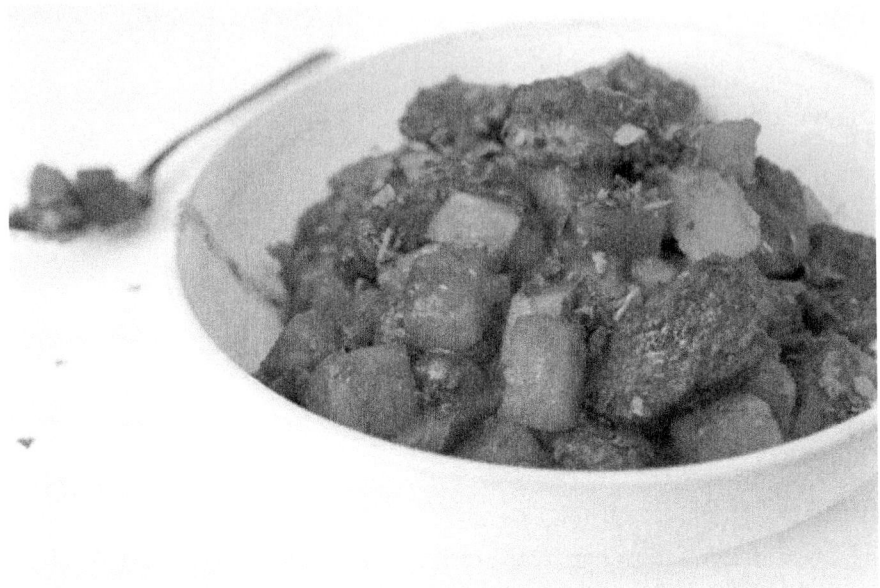

Cooking time: 3-6 hours   **Servings:** 4

Ingredients:

- 1 lb beef stew meat, cut into 1-inch pieces
- 2 tablespoons coconut oil
- 1 onion, chopped
- 1 carrot, chopped
- 1 parsnip, chopped
- 2 oz mushrooms, halved
- 4 cloves garlic, chopped
- ½ teaspoon thyme
- 2 bay leaves
- 2 teaspoon Worcestershire sauce
- 1 cup Guinness stout
- 1 cup beef stock
- 1 teaspoon dried oregano
- fresh parsley
- salt and pepper, to taste

Instructions:

1. Heat oil in a big skillet over medium heat, add beef. Cook for 5-10 minutes stirring constantly until beef is browned from all sides.

2. Transfer beef to a slow cooker.

3. Add onion, carrot, parsnip, mushrooms, garlic, thyme, bay leaves, Worcestershire sauce, Guinness stout, beef stock and oregano. Add salt and pepper to taste.

4. Close the lid and cook on Low for 6 hours or on High for 3-4 hours.

5. Serve topped with parsley.

Nutritional info:

Calories 235; Fats 25g; Net carbs 5g; Protein 12g

Broccoli Beef Soup

Cooking time: 4 hours   **Servings:** 4

Ingredients:

- 1 lb boneless beef chuck, cut into 1-inch pieces
- 1 cup beef broth
- 1 teaspoon sesame oil
- 1 broccoli head, broke into florets
- 1 garlic cloves, minced
- 4 tablespoons soy sauce
- 2 teaspoons brown sugar substitute
- ½ cup water
- 2 tablespoons Xanthan gum

Instructions:

1. Mix beef broth, sesame oil, garlic, soy sauce and sugar in a big bowl.
2. Put beef into slow cooker. Add broth mixture and mix to combine.
3. Close the lid and cook on low for 3-4 hours.
4. Mix water and Xanthan gum in a separate bow. Pour into slow cooker once the time is up.
5. Close the lid and cook on High for another 30 minutes.

Nutritional info:

Calories 370; Fats 31.8g; Net carbs 5.3g; Protein 27g

Creamy Beef Soup

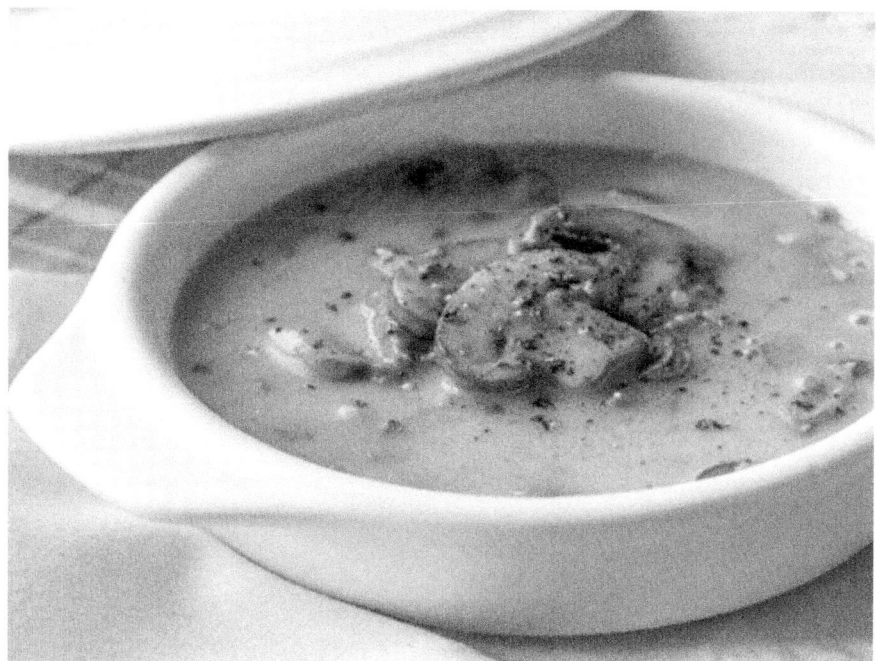

Cooking time: 8-9 hours   **Servings:** 6

Ingredients:

- 1 ½ pound beef rump steak meat, sliced
- 1 pound white mushrooms
- 2 tablespoons ghee
- 1 onion, chopped
- 2 garlic cloves, minced
- 1 ½ quart chicken or vegetable stock
- 1 ½ cup heavy whipping cream
- 1 tablespoon Dijon mustard
- 1 lemon, juice
- 2 teaspoons paprika
- salt, pepper, to taste

Instructions:

1. Heat ghee in a skillet over high heat. Add beef steak pieces and cook until brown.

2. Mix stock, mustard, whipping cream and lemon juice in a bowl.

3. Put browned beef, mushrooms, onion, garlic to the slow cooker.

4. Pour the stock mixture over the meat and veggies. Season with salt, pepper and paprika.

5. Close the lid and cook on Low for 8-9 hours.

Nutritional info:

Calories 424; Fats 34.5 g; Net carbs 6.8g; Protein 28.8g

Beef Bourguignon

Cooking time: 8 hours   **Servings:** 6

Ingredients:

- 1 ½ pound beef roast, sliced
- 1 onion, sliced
- 1 cup carrots, diced
- 2 teaspoons olive oil
- 2 garlic cloves, minced
- ½ teaspoon dried oregano
- ½ teaspoon dried thyme
- 1 teaspoon basil
- 1 tablespoon tomato paste
- 1 cup dry red wine
- salt, pepper, to taste

Instructions:

1. Heat oil in a skillet over medium heat. Add beef slices and cook until brown.
2. Add some oil to the slow cooker and put onion on the bottom. Add garlic.
3. Add beef on top and sprinkle everything with salt, pepper, add oregano, thyme and basil.
4. Add carrots, tomato paste and wine.
5. Close the lid and cook on Low for 8 hours.

Nutritional info:

Calories 276; Fats 18.7 g; Net carbs 5.5g; Protein 25g

Stuffed Bell Peppers

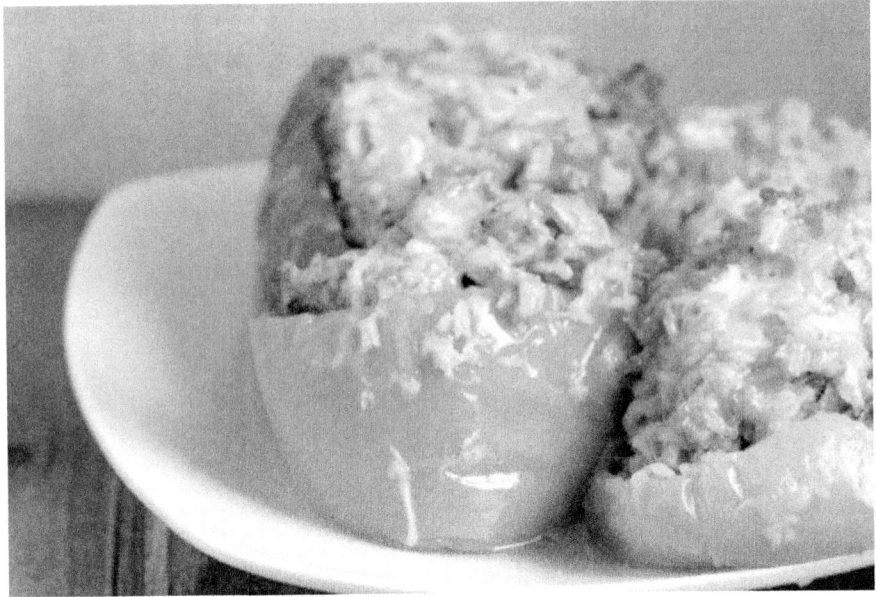

Cooking time: 6-8 hours   **Servings:** 4

Ingredients:

- 4 big bell peppers
- 1 ½ pound ground beef
- 1 onion, chopped
- 2 garlic cloves, chopped
- 7 oz crushed tomatoes

- 2 teaspoons chili powder
- 2 teaspoons ground cumin
- 1/3 cup water
- ½ cup cheese, shredded
- salt, pepper, to taste

Instructions:

1. Heat oil in a skillet over medium heat. Add onion and garlic, sauté for 1-2 minutes.
2. Add beef and cook until brown, for 5-7 minutes.
3. Transfer meat with onion and garlic to a bowl, add crushed tomatoes, chili powder, ground cumin, salt and pepper, mix well.
4. Stuff each bell pepper with beef mixture.

5. Put all stuffed peppers to the slow cooker, add water to the bottom and sprinkle cheese on top of each pepper.

6. Close the lid and cook on Low for 6-8 hours.

Nutritional info:

Calories 210; Fats 18g; Net carbs 7.4g; Protein 14.5g

Beef Cabbage Stir Fry

Cooking time: 3-6 hours   **Servings:** 4

Ingredients:

- 3 cups green cabbage, shredded
- 1 tablespoon olive oil
- 1 pound ground beef
- 1 tablespoon white vinegar
- 1 teaspoon onion powder
- 2 garlic cloves, minced
- 1 tablespoon ginger, fresh, grated
- 1 teaspoon chili flakes
- 7 oz diced tomatoes
- salt, pepper, to taste

Instructions:

1. Mix beef with vinegar, onion powder, garlic, ginger, chili flakes, salt and pepper in a bowl.
2. Add oil to the slow cooker or use a cooking spray.
3. Put 1 ½ cups cabbage of the bottom of the cooker.
4. Put beef on top, add tomatoes and the rest of the cabbage.
5. Close the lid and cook on Low for 5-6 hours or on High for 3 hours.

Nutritional info:

Calories 273; Fats 15.8g; Net carbs 7g; Protein 25.8g

Beef Brisket

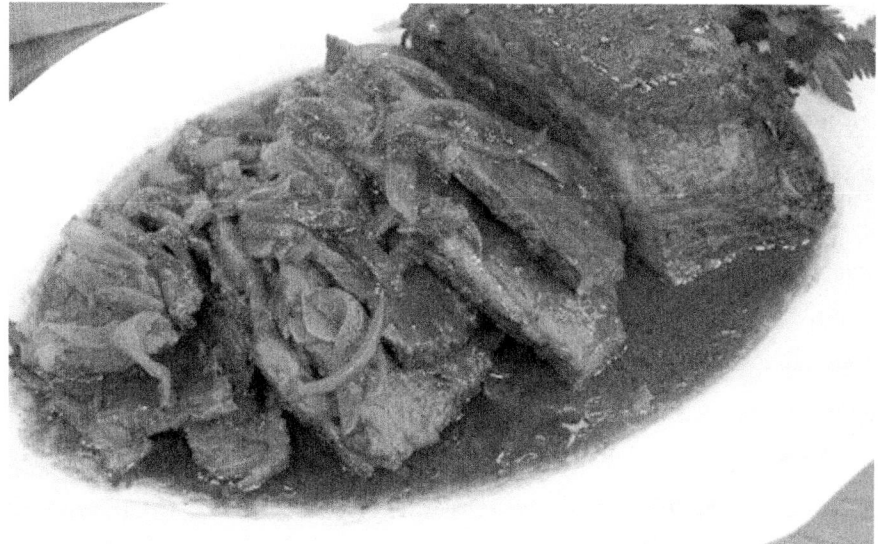

Cooking time: 6-8 hours   **Servings:** 6

Ingredients:

- 2 pounds beef brisket
- 1 pound onions, sliced
- 1 tablespoon olive oil
- 3 garlic cloves, minced
- 2 cups beef broth

- 2 tablespoons Worcestershire sauce
- 1 tablespoon soy sauce
- salt, pepper, to taste

Instructions:

1. Heat oil in a skillet over medium heat. Add onions and cook until slightly brown, for about 4-5 minutes. Add garlic, sauté for 1-2 more minutes.

2. Season the brisket with salt and pepper. Put the seasoned brisket into the slow cooker. Add onion and garlic. Add the sauces and beef broth.

3. Close the lid and cook on Low for 6-8 hours.

Nutritional info:

Calories 353; Fats 22.3g; Net carbs 9.1g; Protein 38.6g

Beef Curry

Cooking time: 6-8 hours   **Servings:** 6

Ingredients:

- 2 pounds beef stew meat, cubed
- 1 onion, chopped
- 2 garlic cloves, chopped
- 1 tablespoon ginger, chopped
- 3 tablespoons curry powder
- 1 cup coconut cream
- 14 oz can diced tomatoes
- 2 tablespoons fresh coriander, chopped
- salt, pepper, to taste

Instructions:

1. Mix coconut cream, ginger, coriander, curry powder, salt and pepper in a slow cooker.
2. Add onion, garlic, tomatoes and beef, mix well.
3. Close the lid and cook on Low for 8-10 hours or on High for 4-6 hours.

Nutritional info:

Calories 409; Fats 29.5g; Net carbs 10.1g; Protein 18.1g

Beef Burgers

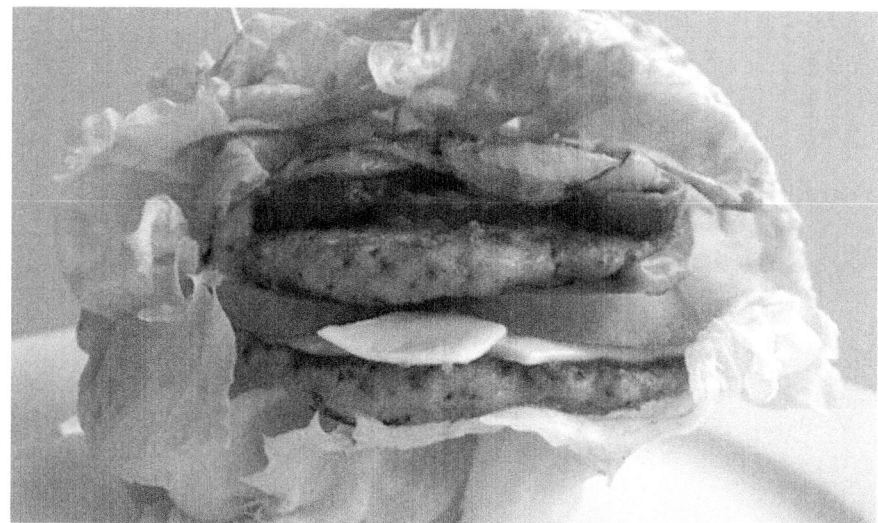

Cooking time: 6-8 hours   **Servings:** 6

Ingredients:

- 2 pounds ground beef
- 2 teaspoons onion powder
- 2 teaspoons garlic powder
- 2 teaspoons paprika
- 1 cup almond meal
- 1 egg
- 2 tablespoons Worcestershire Sauce

- ¼ cup water
- salt, pepper, to taste

For serving:
- lettuce
- tomatoes
- onion
- mustard
- mayonnaise

Instructions:

1. Mix beef, egg, water, almond meal, Worcestershire Sauce, onion powder, garlic powder, paprika, salt and pepper in a bowl.
2. Shape the mixture into 5-6 burger patties, 1-inch thick.

3. Put the patties into the slow cooker, make sure to leave some space between them.

4. Close the lid and cook on Low for 4-6 hours.

5. Serve on lettuce with sliced tomato and onion; top with mayo and mustard.

Nutritional info:

Calories 396; Fats 38.2g; Net carbs 6.2g; Protein 20.5g

Beef Carne Guisada

Cooking time: 6-8 hours   **Servings:** 6

Ingredients:

- 1 ½ pound beef stew meat, cut into cubes
- 1 bay leaf
- 1 tablespoon garlic, minced
- 1 onion, diced
- 1 teaspoon paprika
- 1 teaspoon ground cumin
- salt and pepper, to taste
- 1 teaspoon chili powder
- 1 serrano pepper, minced
- 2 cups broth, chicken or beef
- 1/2 teaspoon oregano
- 1 teaspoon chipotle powder
- 2 tablespoons almond flour

Instructions:

1. Mix almond flower, chipotle powder, oregano, chili powder, ground cumin, paprika, salt and pepper in bowl.
2. Toss the beef pieces with the flour mixture until evenly coated.
3. Put the meat into the slow cooker, add onion, garlic, serrano pepper and broth.
4. Close the lid and cook on Low for 6-8 hours.

Nutritional info:

Calories 250; Fats 28.9g; Net carbs 3.6g; Protein 17g

Kale Ground Beef Keto Style

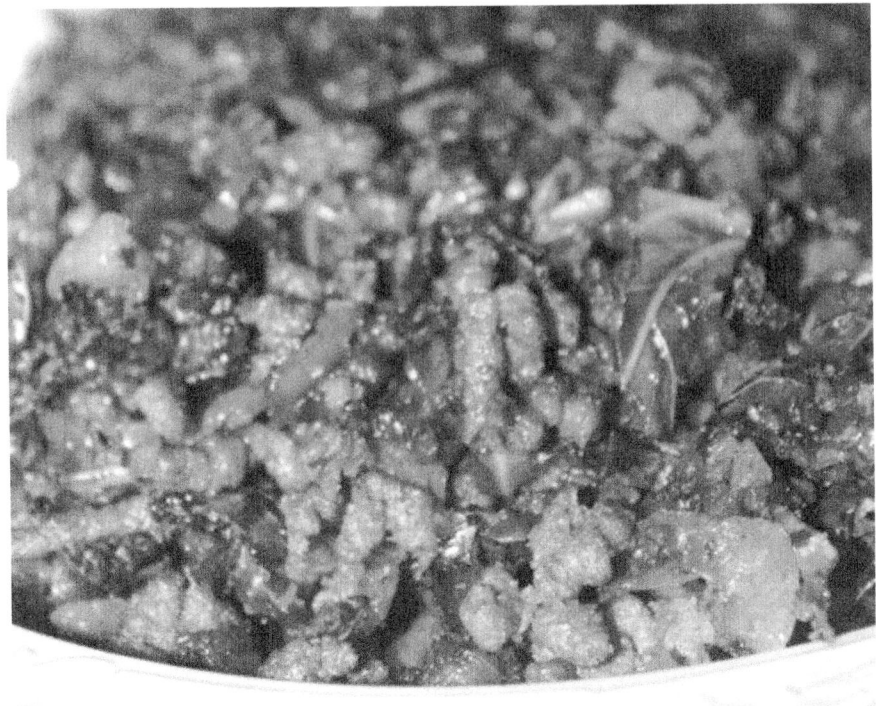

Cooking time: 4-6 hours   **Servings:** 3

Ingredients:

- 11 oz ground beef
- 1 bunch kale
- ½ cup beef broth
- 2 tablespoon cayenne pepper
- 2 tablespoons coconut oil
- 1 tablespoon Chinese five spice powder

- 2 celery ribs, chopped
- ½ onion, chopped
- 5 medium brown mushrooms
- salt and pepper, to taste
- 1 cup water
- 2 tablespoons Xanthan gum

Instructions:

1. Heat oil in a medium pan over high heat. Add ground beef and sauté for 5 minutes. Drain fat and set aside.

2. Clean the pan and heat some more oil in it, add onions and cook for 3 minutes.

3. Put beef, onions, celery ribs, mushrooms and beef broth into a slow cooker. Add cayenne pepper, Chinese five spice powder, salt and pepper to the beef and mix to combine.

4. Close the lid and cook on Low for 6 hours or on High for 4 hours.

5. Meanwhile mix water and Xanthan gum in a separate bowl. Once the beef time is up open the lid and add the mixture. Also add kale.

6. Close the lid and cook for another 30 minutes on Low.

Nutritional info:

Calories 244; Fats 22.2g; Net carbs 6.6g; Protein 16.1g

Pulled Pork

Cooking time: 7-8 hours **Servings:** 5-6

Ingredients:

- 2-3 lbs pork shoulder roast
- 1 cup chicken broth
- 1 onion, sliced
- 2 garlic cloves, minced
- 1 tablespoon Worcestershire sauce
- 1 tablespoon liquid smoke
- ½ teaspoon erythritol or brown sugar Truvia
- 1 teaspoon chili powder
- ½ teaspoon paprika
- ½ teaspoon cumin
- ½ teaspoon garlic powder
- 1 teaspoon salt and black ground pepper

Instructions:

1. Mix erythritol or brown sugar Truvia, chili powder, paprika, cumin, garlic powder, salt and pepper in a bowl.
2. Pat the pork dry with a paper towel. Rub the meat with the spice mixture.
3. Put onion and garlic into the bottom of the Crockpot. Put the pork on top.
4. Mix Worcestershire sauce and liquid smoke in a bowl.
5. Add to the Crockpot, also add broth.
6. Close the lid and cook on Low for 7-8 hours.
7. Take out the meat and pull the pork with fork and knife.
8. Return the meat to the Crockpot, stir a bit and serve.

Nutritional info:

Calories 491; Fats 37.3g; Net carbs 4.8g; Protein 22.2g

Pork with Brussels Sprouts

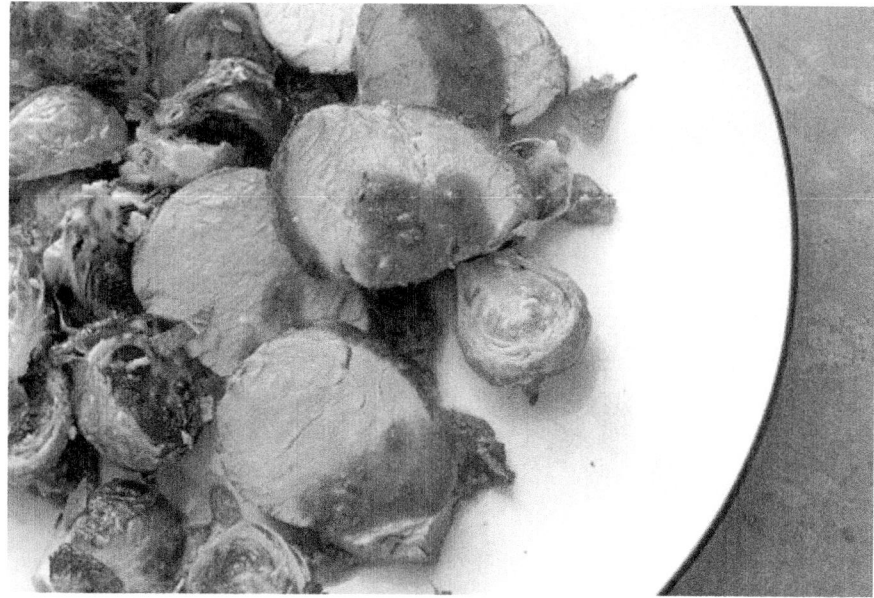

Cooking time: 6 hours   **Servings:** 6

Ingredients:

- 2 pounds pork belly, cubed or sliced
- 1 pound Brussels sprouts
- 2 tablespoons soy sauce
- 1 tablespoon rice vinegar
- 2 garlic cloves, minced
- ½ teaspoon dried thyme
- salt, pepper, to taste

Instructions:

1. Add soy sauce, Brussels sprouts, rice vinegar, garlic and thyme to the slow cooker.
2. Season the meat with salt and pepper, add to the slow cooker.
3. Close the lid and cook on Low for 6 hours.

Nutritional info:

Calories 637; Fats 41g; Net carbs 7.7g; Protein 22.8g

Sweet Lime Ginger Pork

Cooking time: 3-8 hours   **Servings:** 5-6

Ingredients:

- 2 lbs pork loin
- 1 tablespoon olive oil
- ¼ cup soy sauce
- ½ teaspoon erythritol or brown sugar Truvia
- 1 tablespoon Worcestershire Sauce
- 1 lime, juiced
- 2 garlic cloves, minced
- salt, pepper, to taste
- 1 teaspoon fresh ginger, grounded
- 2 tablespoons Xanthan Gum
- 2 tablespoons water

Instructions:

1. Heat oil in a skillet over medium heat. Season pork with salt and pepper, then put it on the hot skillet. Cook for 2-5 minutes both sides.
2. Put the pork into the bottom of the Crockpot.
3. Mix soy sauce, Worcestershire Sauce, erythritol or brown sugar Truvia, lime juice, garlic cloves and ginger in a bowl.
4. Pour the mixture over pork, add water, close the lid and cook on Low for 6-8 hours or on High for 3-5 hours.
5. Transfer the pork to a plate, pour the sauce from the Crockpot to a saucepan.
6. Heat it over medium heat and add Xanthan Gum. Stir until the sauce thickens. Pour over the pork and serve.

Nutritional info:

Calories 223; Fats 22.6g; Net carbs 14.2g; Protein 21.6g

Smoked Pork with Cauliflower Rice

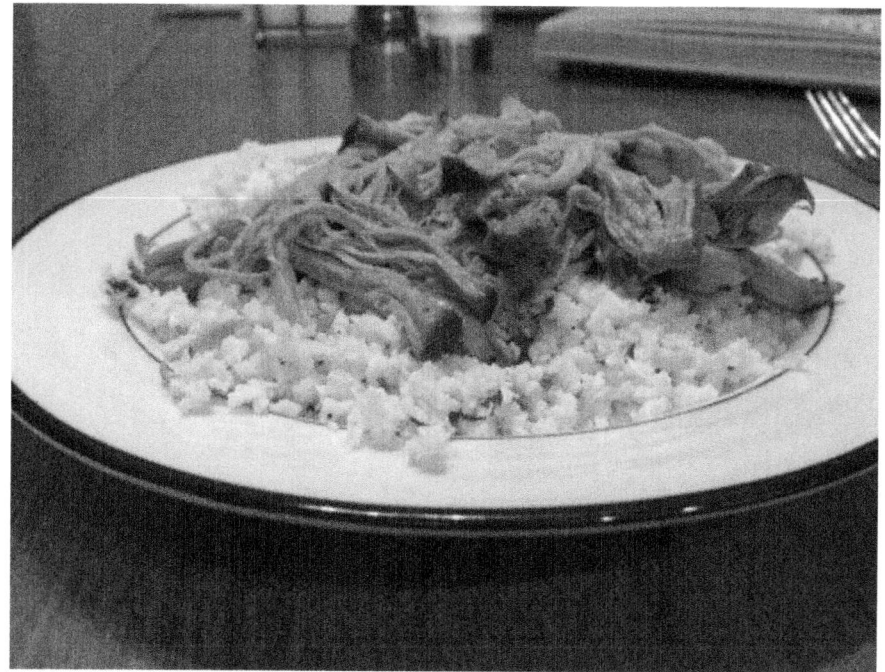

Cooking time: 4-10 hours   **Servings:** 6-7

Ingredients:

- 2 lbs pork roast
- 3 slices nitrate free bacon
- 1 ½ teaspoon sea salt
- 4 garlic cloves, minced

- 1 tablespoon liquid smoke
- 2 cups cauliflower florets
- 2 tablespoons chicken broth
- ½ teaspoon garlic powder

Instructions:

1. Put bacon slices on the bottom of the Crockpot.
2. Rub the pork roast with sea salt (1 teaspoon). Using a knife make several holes in the roast.
3. Put the meat over bacon, fat side down. Add liquid smoke to the Crockpot.

4. Close the lid and cook on High for 4-6 hours, then on Low for 2 hours, or on Low for 8-10 hours.

5. Once the cooking time is up open the lid and shred the meat with a knife and a fork. Stir shredded meat and bacon.

6. To cook the cauliflower rice, steam the florets for 20 minutes, cool them down a bit.

7. Put the florets to the food processor; add broth, sea salt and garlic powder, process until smooth.

8. Serve rice with pulled pork.

Nutritional info:

Calories 309; Fats 25.3g; Net carbs 2.3g; Protein 18.6g

Keto Pork Soup

Cooking time: 3-8 hours **Servings:** 7-8

Ingredients:

- 1 ½ lb pork tenderloin, cubed or cut into stripes
- 1 onion, chopped
- 1 bell pepper, chopped
- 2 garlic cloves, minced
- 1 jalapeno pepper, seeded and chopped
- 1 teaspoon chile powder
- 1 teaspoon cumin
- 5 cups chicken broth
- 1 can diced tomatoes
- salt, pepper, to taste

Instructions:

1. Add pork, onion, bell pepper, jalapeno pepper and garlic to the Crockpot.
2. Season with chile powder, cumin, salt and pepper.
3. Add tomatoes and broth.
4. Close the lid and cook on Low for 6-8 hours or on High for 3-4 hours.

Nutritional info:

Calories 137; Fats 14.1g; Net carbs 6.3g; Protein 8.2g

Curry Pork Stir Fry

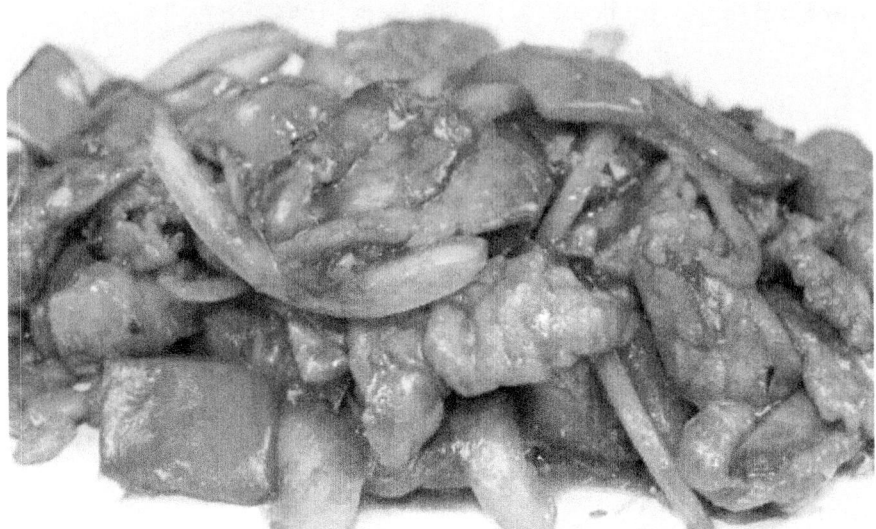

Cooking time: 3-8 hours   **Servings:** 5-6

Ingredients:

- 1.5-2 lbs pork loin, cubed
- 1 cup coconut milk
- 1 ½ medium bell peppers, sliced
- ½ onion, sliced

- 2 garlic cloves, minced
- 1 tablespoon curry powder
- 1 tablespoon Sriracha sauce
- ½ tablespoon olive oil
- salt, pepper, to taste

Instructions:

1. Heat oil in a skillet over medium heat. Season pork cubes with salt and pepper, then put them on the hot skillet. Cook for 3-5 minutes until slightly brown.

2. Put bell peppers, onion and garlic on the bottom of the Crockpot. Add pork cubes on top; add Sriracha sauce, curry powder and coconut milk.

3. Close the lid and cook on Low for 6-8 hours or on High for 3-5 hours.

Nutritional info:

Calories 271; Fats 33.7g; Net carbs 6.7g; Protein 20.6g

Creamy Pork Chops

Cooking time: 3-4 hours   **Servings:** 4

Ingredients:

- 4 big bone-in pork chops
- ½ onion, sliced
- 1 cup heavy whipping cream
- 2 garlic cloves, minced
- 1 oz cream cheese
- 1 tablespoon Italian seasoning
- 1/3 cup chicken or vegetable broth
- 1/3 cup parmesan cheese
- ½ cup cheddar cheese
- salt, pepper, to taste

Instructions:

1. Sprinkle pork chops with salt and pepper.
2. Mix whipping cream, broth, cream cheese, garlic and Italian seasoning in a bowl.
3. Put pork chops into the slow cooker. Add broth mixture, parmesan cheese and cheddar cheese.
4. Close the lid and cook on Low for 3-4 hours.

Nutritional info:

Calories 451; Fats 36.9g; Net carbs 2.9g; Protein 29.2g

Pork Roast

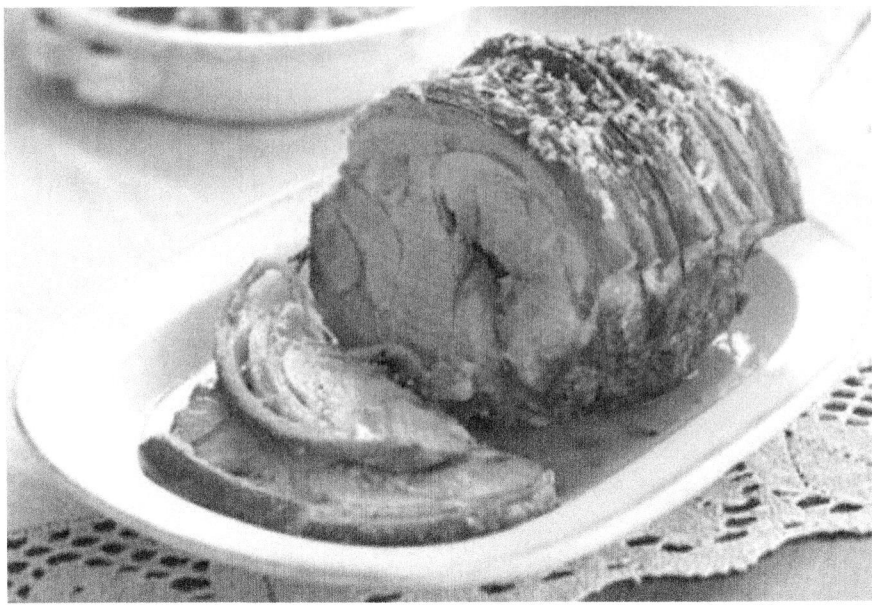

Cooking time: 8 hours   **Servings:** 8

Ingredients:

- 5 pounds pork roast or pork shoulder
- 2 tablespoons fresh rosemary
- 2 tablespoons fresh thyme
- 3 tablespoons dry white wine
- 2 garlic cloves, chopped
- 4 tablespoons olive oil
- 2 bay leaves
- 1 cup water
- salt, pepper, to taste

Instructions:

1. Season meat with salt and pepper. Mix olive oil with rosemary and thyme in a bowl.

2. Pour water into the slow cooker, add meat. Add oil herbs mixture, wine, garlic and bay leaves.

3. Close the lid and cook on Low for 8 hours.

Nutritional info:

Calories 658; Fats 43.9g; Net carbs 1.5g; Protein 31g

Pork Ribs

Cooking time: 4-8 hours   **Servings:** 6

Ingredients:

- 2 pounds pork ribs
- 1 garlic clove, minced
- 1 onion, sliced
- ½ cup water
- salt, pepper, to taste

For Keto BBQ sauce (1 cup):

- 1 cup low-sugar ketchup
- ½ cup chicken bone broth
- ¼ cup apple cider vinegar
- 2 ½ tablespoons erythritol or brown sugar Truvia
- 2 teaspoons paprika
- ½ teaspoon onion powder
- salt and pepper, to taste

Instructions:

1. Season ribs with salt and pepper. Pour water into the slow cooker.
2. Put ribs into the cooker, add onion and garlic.
3. Close the lid and cook on Low for 8 hours or on High for 4 hours.
4. To make BBQ sauce, simply mix all the ingredients in a saucepan, bring to a boil and simmer for 30 minutes.
5. Preheat the oven to 375 F. Put pork ribs on a baking sheet and cover with BBQ sauce and cook for 10-15 minutes.
6. Serve with more sauce and onion from the slow cooker.

Nutritional info:

Calories 351; Fats 30.3g; Net carbs 10.7g; Protein 21.4g

Pork Tenderloin

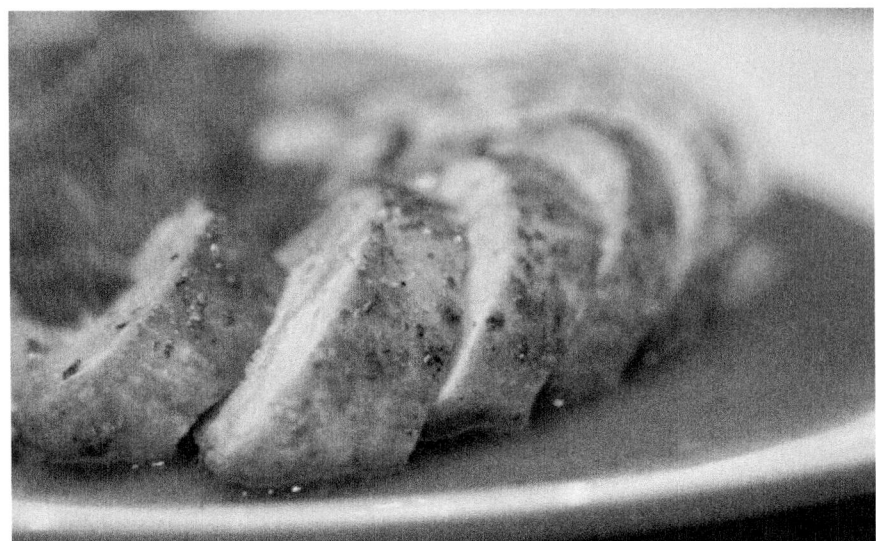

Cooking time: 3-6 hours   **Servings:** 4

Ingredients:

- 1 pound pork tenderloin
- 1 tablespoon olive oil
- 2 garlic cloves, minced
- ¼ cup balsamic vinegar
- 1 tablespoon coconut aminos
- ½ tablespoon Worcestershire sauce
- salt, black pepper, to taste

Instructions:

1. Add olive oil and garlic to the Crockpot.
2. Mix vinegar, coconut aminos, and Worcestershire sauce in a bowl.
3. Season tenderloin with salt and pepper.
4. Put pork tenderloin into the Crockpot, pour the sauce mixture on top.
5. Close the lid and cook on Low for 5-6 hours or on High for 3-4 hours.

Nutritional info:

Calories 188; Fats 15.8g; Net carbs 1.3g; Protein 20.3g

Lamb Chops

Cooking time: 6-8 hours **Servings:** 6

Ingredients:

- 2 ½ pounds lamb chops
- 1 onion, sliced
- 3 garlic cloves, minced
- 2 tablespoons fresh rosemary
- 2 tablespoons cooking red wine
- salt, black pepper, to taste

Instructions:

1. Put sliced onions on the bottom of the slow cooker.
2. Add chops on top, add garlic, wine, salt, pepper and rosemary.
3. Close the lid and cook on Low for 6-8 hours.

Nutritional info:

Calories 369; Fats 34.1g; Net carbs 3g; Protein 23.4g

Sweet Pork Loin

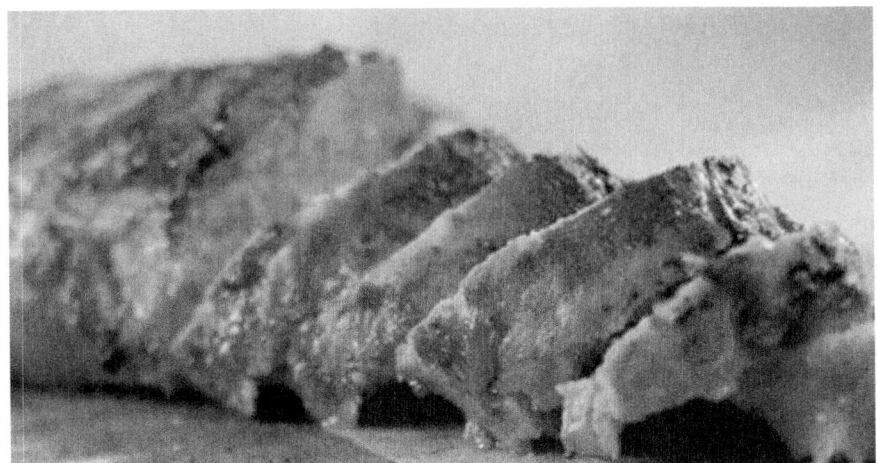

Cooking time: 8-10 hours   **Servings:** 8

Ingredients:

- 4 pounds bone-in pork loin roast
- 1 tablespoon Dijon mustard
- 1 tablespoon balsamic vinegar
- 2 garlic cloves, peeled
- 2/3 cup erythritol or brown sugar Truvia
- ¼ teaspoon cinnamon
- salt, pepper, to taste

Instructions:

1. Season pork roast with salt and pepper.
2. Mix mustard, sweetener, cinnamon and vinegar in a bowl. Rub the roast with the mustard mixture.
3. Close the lid and cook on Low for 8-10 hours.

Nutritional info:

Calories 594; Fats 34.1g; Net carbs 8.3g; Protein 16.9g

Keto Sweet Maple Lamb

Cooking time: 7 hours   **Servings:** 6

Ingredients:

- 2 pounds lamb leg
- 3 garlic cloves, minced
- 3 sprigs thyme
- ½ teaspoon dried or fresh rosemary
- 2 tablespoons Dijon mustard

- 4 tablespoons olive oil
- 1 cup water
- 1 cup erythritol
- 1 ½ tablespoon Maple extract
- ½ teaspoon Xantham gum
- salt, pepper, to taste

Instructions:

1. Prepare the Keto Maple Syrup first: mix water, erythritol and Maple extract in a saucepan.
2. Bring to a boil and stir for 4-5 minutes until erythritol dissolves.
3. Pour the mixture to a blender, add half of Xantham gum and puree. Add the remaining Xantham gum and puree again. If the syrup is not thick enough, you can add more Xantham gum.
4. Take the lamb leg, season it with salt, pepper, rub with oil, mustard and 1 tablespoon of the home made Maple Syrup.
5. Add garlic, thyme and rosemary into the slow cooker.
6. Close the lid and cook on Low for 7 hours.

Nutritional info:

Calories 274; Fats 35.2g; Net carbs 1.6g; Protein 27.5g

Lamb Stew

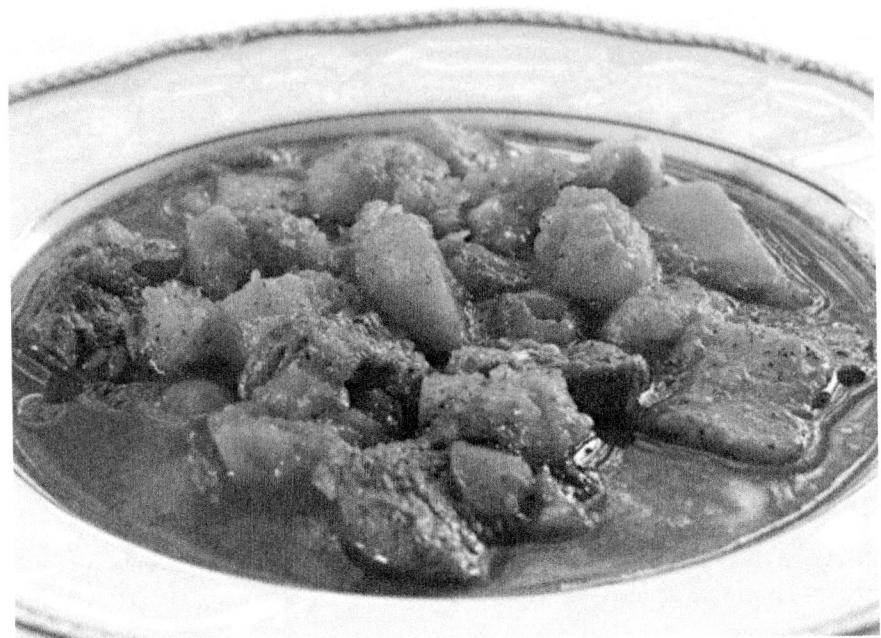

Cooking time: 3-6 hours   **Servings:** 6

Ingredients:

- 2 pounds lamb leg, cubed
- 1 onion, sliced
- 3 carrots, sliced
- 3 garlic cloves, minced
- 14 oz beef broth
- ¼ cup red wine
- salt, pepper, to taste

Instructions:

1. Add lamb meat, onion, carrots, garlic into the slow cooker.
2. Pour beef broth and wine into the cooker, season with salt and pepper.
3. Close the lid and cook on Low for 6 hours or on High for 3 hours.

Nutritional info:

Calories 241; Fats 27.1g; Net carbs 5.7g; Protein 12.6g

Lamb Vegetable Soup

Cooking time: 4-8 hours   **Servings:** 4

Ingredients:

- 3 lamb shanks
- 1 cauliflower head, cut into florets
- 1 onion, cubed
- 1 carrot, cubed
- 1 stalk celery, cubed
- 4 cups beef stock
- salt, pepper, to taste

Instructions:

1. Add lamb, onion, carrot, celery and cauliflower into the slow cooker.
2. Pour beef broth into the cooker, season with salt and pepper.
3. Close the lid and cook on Low for 8 hours or on High for 4 hours.

Nutritional info:

Calories 151; Fats 15.4g; Net carbs 8.6g; Protein 12.8g

North African Lamb Soup

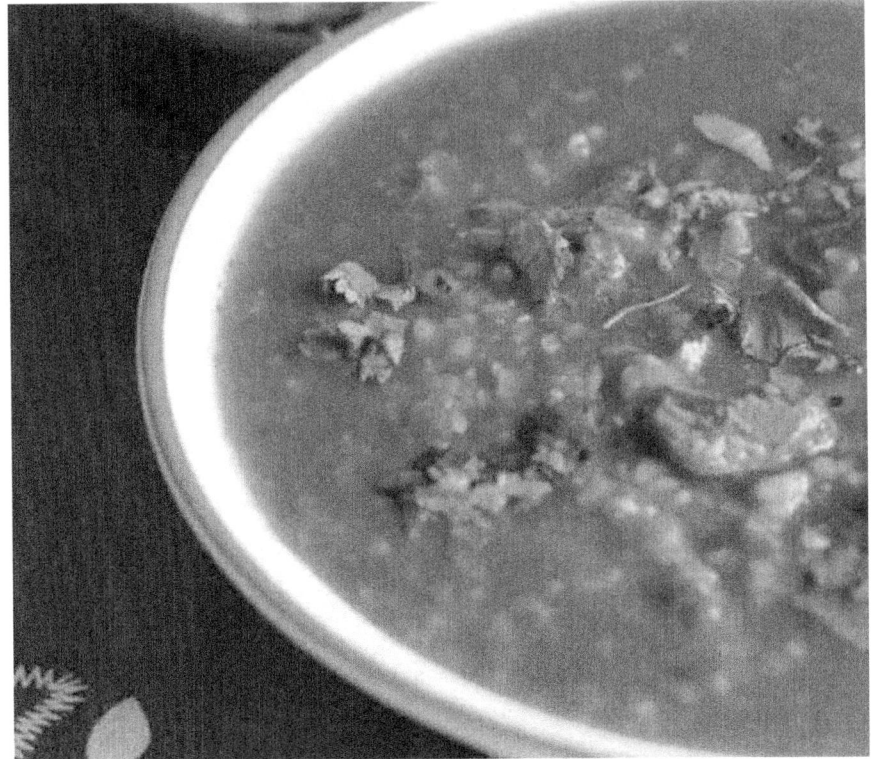

Cooking time: 1-6 hours   **Servings:** 4

Ingredients:

- 1 pound ground lamb
- 3 oz dried apricots, chopped
- 2 tablespoons olive oil
- 1 stalk celery, chopped
- 1 bell pepper, chopped
- ½ can (7 oz) diced tomatoes
- 2 garlic cloves, minced

- 2 teaspoons ground cinnamon
- 2 teaspoons ground cumin
- 2 teaspoons paprika
- 1 lemon, juiced
- 10 oz water
- 1 teaspoon erythritol
- salt, pepper, to taste

Instructions:

1. Soak apricots in water for 1-2 hours, drain.

2. Heat oil in a skillet over medium heat. Add ground lamb and cook for 2-3 minutes until slightly brown.

3. Add apricots, celery, bell pepper and diced tomatoes into the slow cooker.

4. Add water, lemon juice to the cooker, add garlic, ground cinnamon, ground cumin, paprika, erythritol, salt and pepper.

5. Close the lid and cook on Low for 4-6 hours or on High for 1-2 hours.

Nutritional info:

Calories 326; Fats 28.8g; Net carbs 10.1g; Protein 16.3g

Lamb Bone Broth

Cooking time: 24-30 hours   **Servings:** 4

Ingredients:

- 1 pound lamb bones
- 1 onion, diced
- 1 carrot, diced
- 1 stalk celery, chopped
- 2 garlic cloves, minced
- 3 sprigs rosemary
- 3 sprigs thyme
- 10 cups water
- salt, pepper, to taste

Instructions:

1. Preheat the oven to 400F. Place the lamb bones on a baking sheet, cook for 30-40 minutes.
2. Add onion, carrot, celery, garlic and cooked lamb bones to the slow cooker.
3. Add rosemary, thyme, salt, pepper and water to the cooker.
4. Close the lid and cook on Low for 24-30 hours.
5. Strain the broth through a fine meshed sieve and transfer it into jars.
6. Refrigerate the broth. Once cooled, remove the fat layer (or you can leave some).

Nutritional info:

Calories 236; Fats 18.6g; Net carbs 5.8g; Protein 12.5g

Lamb Curry

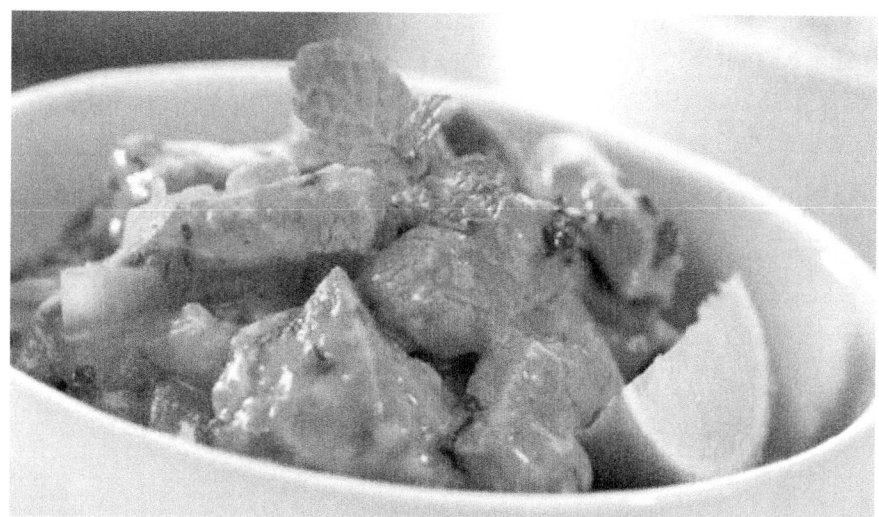

Cooking time: 6 hours   **Servings:** 7

Ingredients:

- 2 pounds lamb shoulder, diced
- 2 teaspoons olive oil
- 3 tablespoons Ghee
- 1 onion, diced
- 1 cup heavy cream
- 2 teaspoons ginger, chopped
- 3 garlic cloves, minced
- 1 teaspoon ground cinnamon
- 1 teaspoon onion powder
- 1 teaspoon Kashmiri Chili Powder
- 2 teaspoons ground cumin
- 2 teaspoons coriander
- 1 teaspoon ground cardamom
- 1 teaspoon paprika
- ½ cup almonds, flaked
- 1 cup coconut milk
- salt, pepper, to taste

Instructions:

1. Mix ginger, garlic, cumin, coriander, onion powder, cardamom, paprika, Kashmiri Chili Powder and olive oil in a bowl.
2. Add the lamb meat and mix well, marinate for 1 hour in a fridge.

3. Heat oil in a skillet over medium heat. Brown lamb meat for 2-3 minutes.

4. Add lamb, Ghee, onion, heavy cream, almonds, coconut milk, salt and pepper to the slow cooker.

5. Close the lid and cook on Low for 6 hours.

Nutritional info:

Calories 480; Fats 38g; Net carbs 2g; Protein 30g

Indian Lamb Stew

Cooking time: 6-8 hours   **Servings:** 6

Ingredients:

- 2 lbs lamb shoulder, cubed
- 2 onions, chopped
- 1 apple, chopped
- 2 celery stalks, chopped
- 1 red chili pepper, chopped
- 2 garlic cloves, minced
- 1 can 14 oz diced tomatoes
- 2 tablespoons curry powder
- 4 tablespoons coconut oil
- 4 tablespoons water
- salt, pepper, to taste

Instructions:

1. Put lamb meat, onions, apple, celery, red chili pepper and garlic into the slow cooker.
2. Season with salt, pepper and curry powder.
3. Add water, oil and diced tomatoes.
4. Close the lid and cook on Low for 8 hours or on High for 6 hours.

Nutritional info:

Calories 407; Fats 30.6g; Net carbs 11.3g; Protein 23.5g

Herbed Lamb Shanks

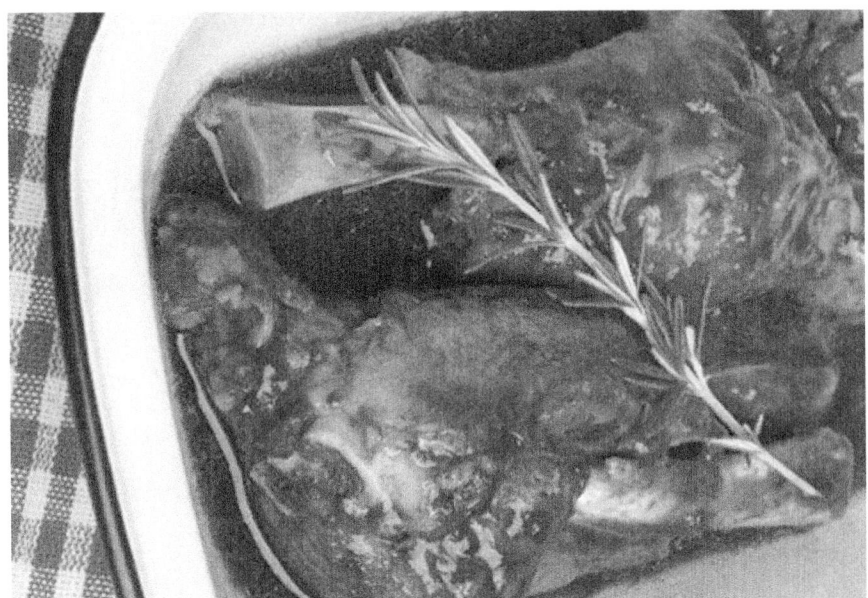

Cooking time: 6-8 hours   **Servings:** 6

Ingredients:

- 2 lbs lamb shoulder, cubed
- 2 onions, chopped
- 1 apple, chopped
- 2 celery stalks, chopped
- 1 red chili pepper, chopped
- 2 garlic cloves, minced

- 1 can 14 oz diced tomatoes
- 2 tablespoons curry powder
- 4 tablespoons coconut oil
- 4 tablespoons water
- salt, pepper, to taste

Instructions:

1. Put lamb meat, onions, apple, celery, red chili pepper and garlic into the slow cooker.
2. Season with salt, pepper and curry powder.
3. Add water, oil and diced tomatoes.

4. Close the lid and cook on Low for 8 hours or on High for 6 hours.

Nutritional info:

Calories 407; Fats 30.6g; Net carbs 11.3g; Protein 23.5g

Moroccan Lamb Chops

Cooking time: 6-8 hours   **Servings:** 6

Ingredients:

- 2 ½ pounds lamb chops
- 2 tablespoons Moroccan spice mix (Ras el Hanout)
- ½ cup beef stock
- ¼ cup olive oil
- 2 tablespoons lemon juice
- ¼ cup fresh parsley, chopped
- 2 tablespoons fresh mint, chopped
- ½ teaspoon smoked paprika
- 1 teaspoon red pepper flakes
- 3 garlic cloves, chopped
- 2 tablespoons lemon zest
- salt, pepper, to taste

Instructions:

1. Pour stock into the slow cooker. Season lamb chops with salt, pepper and Ras el Hanout.

2. Add chops to the slow cooker and close the lid.

3. Cook on low for 6-8 hours. You can also fry the chops a bit before slow cooking (1-2 minutes on each side).

4. Blend the ingredients for the Charmoula sauce: oil, lemon juice, parsley, fresh mint, smoked paprika, pepper flakes, garlic, lemon zest, salt and pepper. The sauce should look like pesto.

5. Serve lamb chops with the Charmoula sauce.

Nutritional info:

Calories 440; Fats 32.5g; Net carbs 2.3g; Protein 23.7g

Rack of Lamb

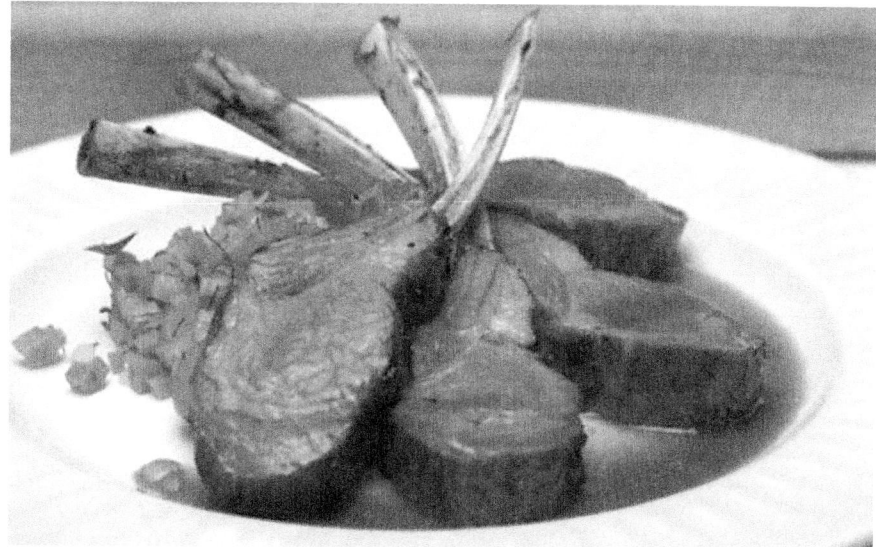

Cooking time: 6-8 hours   **Servings:** 8

Ingredients:

- 2 pounds rack lamb
- 3 tablespoons olive oil
- 1 cup red wine
- 2 tablespoons fresh rosemary
- 1 tablespoon fresh thyme

- 3 garlic cloves, minced
- 1 teaspoon lemon zest
- 1 teaspoon ginger, minced
- salt, pepper, to taste

Instructions:

1. Heat oil in a skillet over medium heat. Brown rack lamb on each side for 2-3 minutes.
2. Mix red wine, rosemary, thyme, garlic, lemon zest, ginger, salt and pepper in a bowl.
3. Put the rack lamb to the slow cooker; pour the wine mixture on top.
4. Close the lid and cook on Low for 6-8 hours
5. Serve with juices from your Crockpot.

Nutritional info:

Calories 266; Fats 25.4g; Net carbs 2.1g; Protein 13.2g

Broccoli and Tofu Curry

Cooking Time: 4 hours   **Servings:** 3

Ingredients:

- 1 cup firm Tofu
- 6 oz light coconut milk
- 1 tablespoon curry powder
- 1 tablespoon Garam Masala
- 1 garlic clove, minced
- ½ broccoli head, broke into florets
- ½ onion, chopped
- 1 tablespoon unsweetened peanut butter

Instructions:

1. Blend onion, garlic, peanut butter and coconut milk in a food processor. Add curry powder, Garam Masala, salt if needed. Mix to combine.

2. Pour the mixture into a zip lock bag and add tofu and broccoli to it. Mix and make sure tofu and broccoli are coated well.

3. Put tofu and broccoli into a slow cooker, add the sauce mixture.

4. Close the lid and cook on Low for 4 hours.

Nutritional info:

Calories 240; Fats 21g; Net carbs 8g; Protein 15g

Italian Tomato Basil Soup

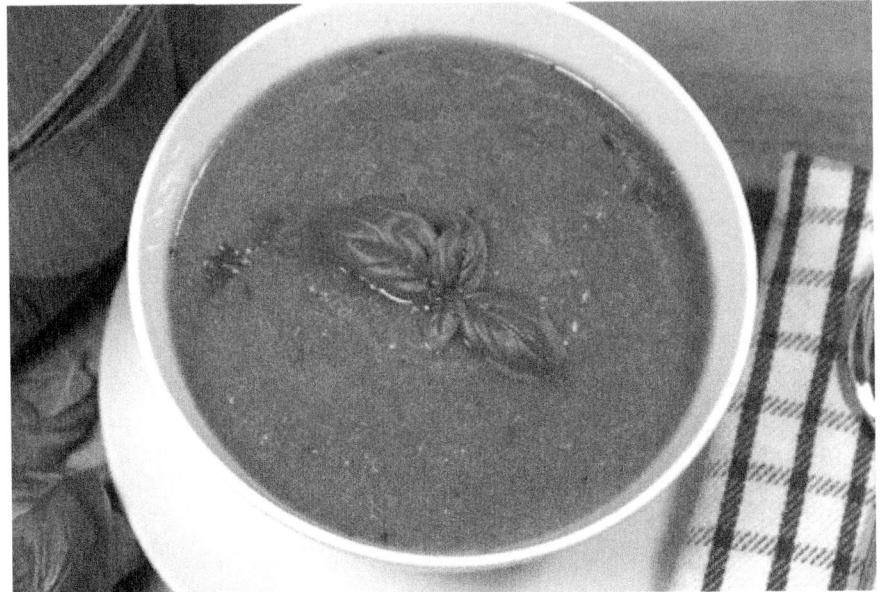

Cooking Time: 3-7 hours   **Servings:** 6-7

Ingredients:

- 7 oz Roma tomatoes
- ½ cup basil leaves, chopped
- 4 cups vegetable broth
- 1 cup carrots, diced
- 1 cup yellow onions, diced
- 4 garlic cloves, minced
- 1 tablespoon olive oil
- 2 bay leaves
- 1 teaspoon erythritol or brown sugar Truvia
- ¾ cup heavy cream
- salt, pepper, to taste

Instructions:

1. Heat oil in a skillet over medium heat. Add carrots, onion and garlic, sauté for 2-3 minutes.

2. Put vegetables to the Crockpot. Add tomatoes, basil leaves, bay leaves, broth and erythritol or brown sugar Truvia.

3. Close the lid and cook on Low for 6-7 hours or on High for 3-4 hours.

4. Once the cooking timer is up open the lid and discard bay leaves. Pour the soup mixture to a food processor and blend until smooth.

5. Return it to the Crockpot, add heavy cream, salt and pepper, stir the soup on Low for 15-20 minutes.

6. You may add some water if you find the soup too thick.

Nutritional info:

Calories 135; Fats 9.6g; Net carbs 8g; Protein 3.9g

Spaghetti Squash

Cooking Time: 4-6 hours   **Servings:** 4

Ingredients:

- 1 whole spaghetti squash
- 1 ½ cups water
- ½ cup Parmesan cheese, grated

Instructions:

1. Wash spaghetti squash thoroughly.

2. Put it into the Crockpot, add water.

3. Close the lid and cook on Low for 4-6 hours.

4. Remove spaghetti squash from the Crockpot, let it rest for 15-20 minutes.

5. Halve it lengthwise and remove seeds. Shred with a fork and serve with grated Parmesan on top.

Nutritional info:

Calories 86; Fats 4.5g; Net carbs 3.8g; Protein 4.8g

Vegetable Bolognese with Zucchini Noodles

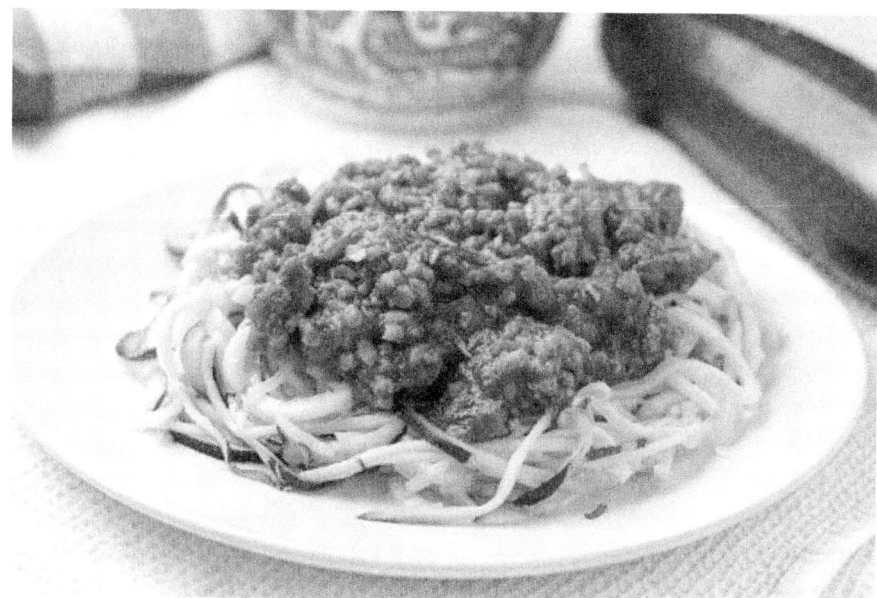

Cooking Time: 3-4 hours   **Servings:** 5

Ingredients:

- 1 cauliflower head, cut into florets
- 4-5 zucchinis cut into thin, noodle-like strips
- ¾ cup red onion, diced
- 2 garlic cloves, minced
- 1 can diced tomatoes, no salt added
- 1 teaspoon dried basil flakes
- 1 teaspoon oregano flakes
- ½ cup vegetable broth
- salt, pepper, to taste

Instructions:

1. Add cauliflower florets, onion, garlic and tomatoes to the Crockpot.
2. Season with salt, pepper, add dried basil flakes, oregano flakes and broth.
3. Close the lid and cook on High for 3-4 hours.

4. Open the lid and smash the cauliflower with a fork until the florets break up.

5. Now cook zucchini noodles. Bring a medium pot of water to a boil, add noodles and cook for 1 minute.

6. Drain and rinse with cold water.

7. Serve Bolognese sauce over noodles.

Nutritional info:

Calories 53; Fats 4.5g; Net carbs 8.5g; Protein 3.5g

Cheesy Risotto

Cooking Time: 2-2.5 hours   **Servings:** 4

Ingredients:

- 1 cauliflower head florets, riced
- 1 onion, chopped
- 2 garlic cloves, minced
- 1 tablespoon olive oil
- 1 cup vegetable broth
- 1 cup Cheddar cheese, shredded
- 1 cup parmesan cheese, grated
- 4 sprigs fresh thyme
- salt, pepper, to taste

Instructions:

1. Heat oil in a skillet over medium heat. Add onions and sauté for 1-2 minutes until translucent. Add garlic and cook for 1 more minute.
2. Add cauliflower rice, cook for 2 more minutes.
3. Transfer vegetables to the Crockpot. Add broth, thyme, salt and pepper.
4. Close the lid and cook on High for 2-2.5 hours.
5. Once the cooking timer is up, open the lid and stir in Cheddar cheese and parmesan cheese. Cook on Low for 15 more minutes.

Nutritional info:

Calories 243; Fats 17.8g; Net carbs 6.3g; Protein 15g

Keto Falafel

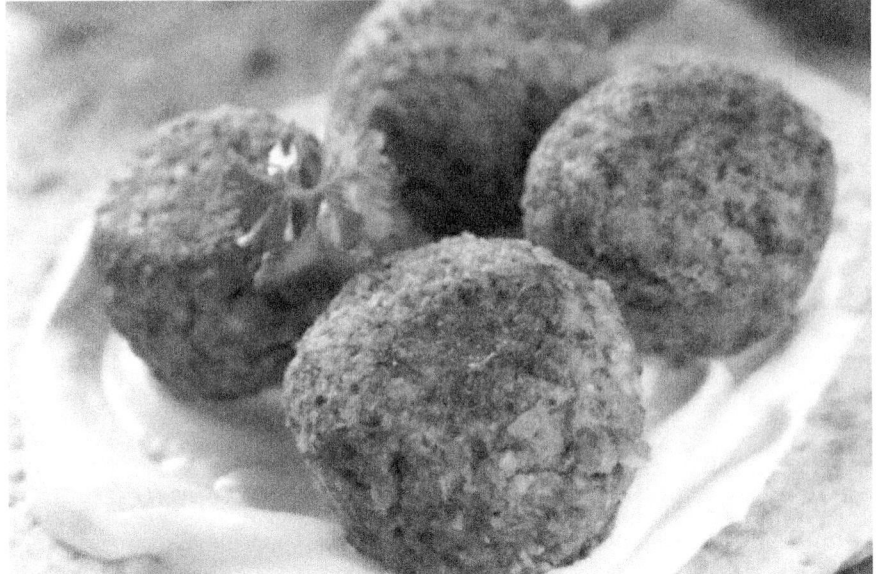

Cooking Time: 2-5 hours   **Servings:** 4-5

Ingredients:

- 1 cup cauliflower head florets, pureed
- ½ cup almonds, grounded
- 1 garlic clove, minced
- 1 medium egg
- 3 tablespoon coconut flour

- 1 tablespoon ground coriander
- ½ teaspoon cayenne pepper
- 1 teaspoon ground cumin
- 2 tablespoons olive oil
- salt, pepper, to taste

Instructions:

1. Mix pureed cauliflower with almonds in a bowl. Add egg, garlic, coconut flour, ground coriander, cayenne pepper, ground cumin, salt and pepper. Stir well to combine.

2. Form medium sized patties of falafel. Add olive oil to the Crockpot.

3. Put falafels to the Crockpot, close the lid and cook on High for 2-5 hours.

Nutritional info:

Calories 281; Fats 24g; Net carbs 5g; Protein 8g

Minestrone Soup

Cooking time: 3-6 hours   **Servings:** 3

Ingredients:

- 1 can black soy beans
- 35 oz vegetable broth
- 2 tablespoons olive oil
- ½ onion, chopped
- ½ celery, diced
- 1 garlic clove, minced
- 6 oz tomato paste
- 2 bay leaves
- 1 fresh rosemary sprig
- 1 tablespoon fresh basil, chopped
- 1 tablespoon fresh parsley, chopped
- 1 zucchini, diced
- 1 cup spinach, chopped
- salt, pepper, to taste
- parmesan cheese, grated

Instructions:

1. Put beans and half of vegetable broth into a food processor and blend well.
2. Heat oil in a medium pan over high heat. Add onion, celery and garlic and cook for 15 minutes stirring constantly.
3. Pour beans and broth mixture into a slow cooker. Add remaining broth, bay leaves, paste, parmesan cheese, vegetables from the pan, salt and pepper.
4. Add rosemary, basil and parsley. Close the lid and cook on Low for 5 hours or on High for 2 hours.
5. After the time is up add zucchini and spinach. Cook for another 1 hour on Low or High.
6. Serve topped with parmesan, remove bay leaves.

Nutritional info:

Calories 304; Fats 16.9g; Net carbs 9.9g; Protein 19.3g

Spinach Soup

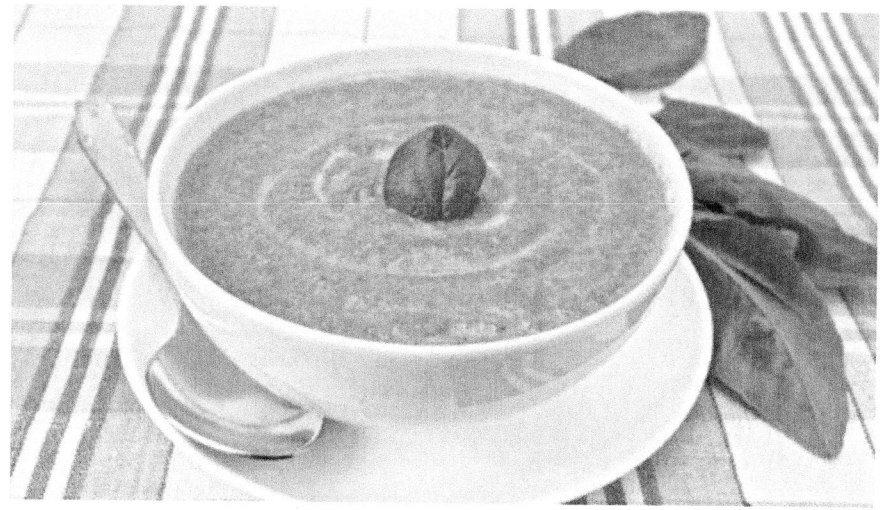

Cooking time: 6-8 hours   **Servings:** 4

Ingredients:

- 2 pounds spinach
- ¼ cup cream cheese
- 1 onion, diced
- 2 cups heavy cream
- 1 garlic clove, minced
- 2 cups water
- salt, pepper, to taste

Instructions:

1. Pour water into the slow cooker. Add spinach, salt and pepper.
2. Add cream cheese, onion, garlic and heavy cream.
3. Close the lid and cook on Low for 6-8 hours.
4. Puree soup with blender and serve.

Nutritional info:

Calories 322; Fats 28.2g; Net carbs 10.1g; Protein 12.2g

Mashed Cauliflower with Herbs

Cooking time: 3-6 hours   **Servings:** 4

Ingredients:

- 1 cauliflower head, cut into florets
- 3 garlic cloves, peeled
- ½ teaspoon fresh rosemary, chopped
- ½ teaspoon fresh thyme, chopped
- ½ teaspoon fresh sage, chopped
- ½ teaspoon fresh parsley, chopped
- 1 cup vegetable broth
- 5 cups water
- 3 tablespoons ghee
- salt, pepper, to taste

Instructions:

1. Pour broth into the slow cooker, add cauliflower florets.
2. Add water, it should cover cauliflower.
3. Close the lid and cook on Low for 6 hours or on High for 3 hour.
4. Once cooked, drain water from the slow cooker.
5. Add herbs, salt, pepper and ghee, puree with a blender.

Nutritional info:

Calories 115; Fats 12g; Net carbs 4.7g; Protein 6.2g

Kale Quiche

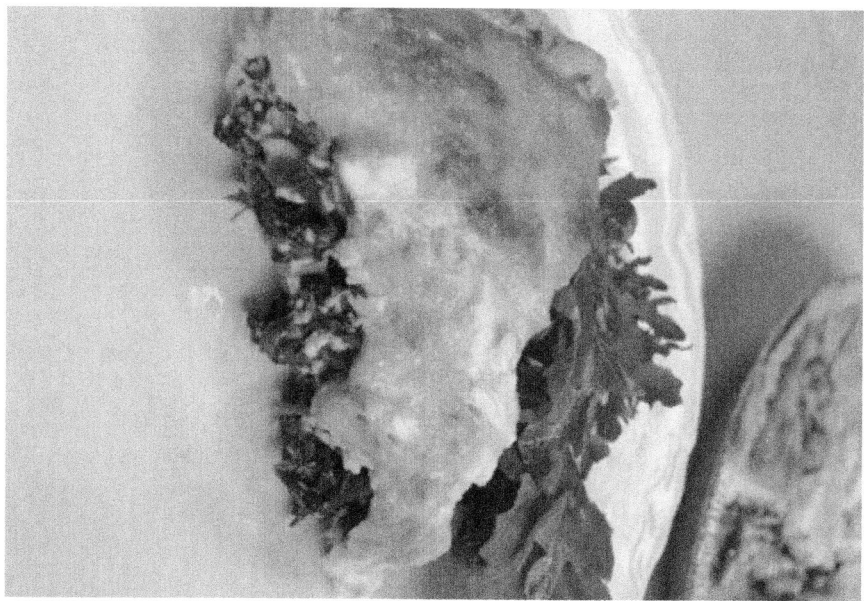

Cooking Time: 3-5 hours   **Servings:** 3

Ingredients:

- 1 cup almond milk
- 6 eggs
- 1 cup CarbQuick Baking Mix
- 2 cups spinach, chopped
- ½ bell pepper, chopped
- 3 cups fresh baby kale, chopped
- 1 teaspoon garlic, chopped
- 1/3 cup fresh basil, chopped
- salt, pepper, to taste
- 1 tablespoon olive oil

Instructions:

1. Add oil to a slow cooker or use a cooking spray.

2. Beat eggs into a slow cooker; add almond milk and CarbQuick Baking Mix, mix to combine.

3. Add spinach, bell pepper, garlic and basil, stir to combine.

4. Close the lid and cook on Low for 5 hours or on High for 3 hours.

5. Make sure the quiche is done, check the center with a toothpick, it should be dry.

Nutritional info:

Calories 273; Fats 24.4g; Net carbs 5.8g; Protein 10.5g

Vegan Frittata with Feta and Artichoke Hearts

Cooking Time: 3 hours   **Servings:** 4

Ingredients:

- 14 oz (1 can) artichoke hearts, drained
- 12 oz (1 can) roasted red peppers, drained
- 1/3 cup green onions, chopped
- 8 eggs
- 4 oz Feta cheese, crumbled
- salt, pepper, to taste
- ¼ cup parsley, chopped
- 2 tablespoons olive oil

Instructions:

1. Add oil to a slow cooker. Put artichoke hearts on the bottom, add roasted red peppers and green onions.

2. Beat eggs to combine yolks and whites well. Pour eggs into slow cooker over vegetables and stir gently.

3. Add salt and pepper, also you can add some dried thyme or rosemary. Sprinkle eggs and vegetables with Feta.

4. Close the lid and cook on Low for 2-3 hours. The cheese should melt and the eggs should be firm.

5. Serve topped with parsley.

Nutritional info:

Calories 332; Fats 22.1g; Net carbs 8.1g; Protein 19.3g

Spinach Stuffed Portobello

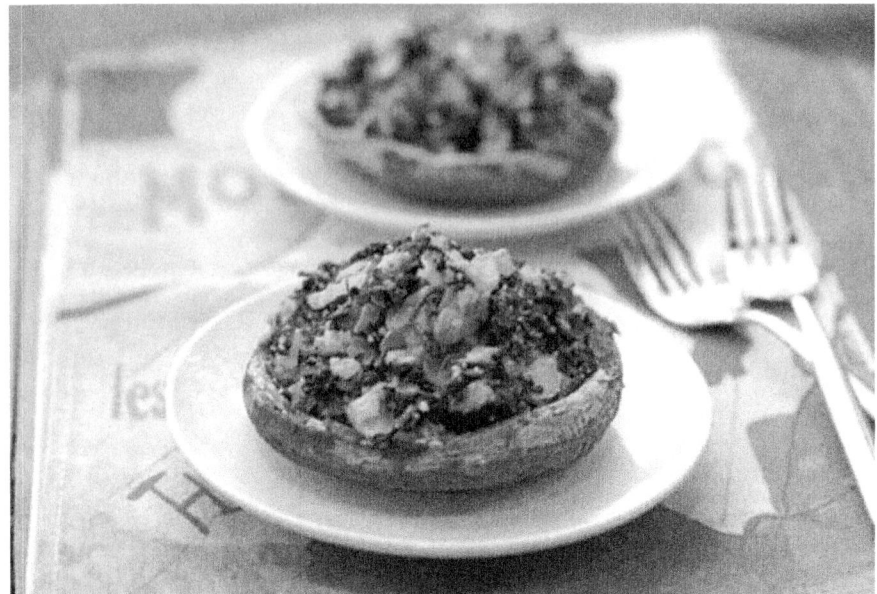

Cooking time: 3 hours **Servings:** 8

Ingredients:

- 12 oz medium sized Portobello mushrooms, stems removed
- 3 tablespoons olive oil
- ½ onion, chopped
- 2 cups fresh spinach, rinsed and chopped
- 3 garlic cloves, minced
- 1 cup chicken broth
- 3 tablespoons parmesan cheese, grated
- 1/3 teaspoon dried thyme
- salt, pepper, to taste

Instructions:

1. Heat oil in a medium pan over high heat. Add onion, cook until translucent stirring constantly. Add spinach and thyme, cook for 1-2 minutes until spinach is wilted.

2. Brush each mushroom with olive oil.

3. Put 1 tablespoon of onion and spinach stuffing into each mushroom.

4. Pour chicken broth into slow cooker. Put stuffed mushrooms on the bottom.

5. Close the lid and cook on High for 3 hours.

6. Once cooked, sprinkle mushrooms with parmesan cheese and serve.

Nutritional info:

Calories 310g; Fats 21g; Net carbs 3g; Protein 12g

Herbed Vegetable Soup

Cooking time: 4-8 hours   **Servings:** 6

Ingredients:

- ½ can of 14 oz diced tomatoes
- 1 ½ cups vegetable broth
- 5 oz mushrooms, fresh or canned
- 1 onion, chopped
- 2 garlic cloves, minced
- 1 zucchini, thinly sliced
- ½ cauliflower head, broken into florets
- 1 teaspoon dried basil
- 1 packet sugar substitute
- salt, pepper, to taste
- 1 tablespoon mozzarella cheese, grated

Instructions:

1. Put tomatoes, mushrooms, onion, garlic, zucchini and cauliflower into slow cooker.
2. Add salt, pepper, basil and vegetable broth.
3. Close the lid and cook on Low for 8 hours or on High for 4 hours.
4. Serve topped with mozzarella cheese.

Nutritional info:

Calories 125g; Fats 15g; Net carbs 2.1g; Protein 11.9g

Cauliflower Pizza with Low Carb Alfredo Sauce

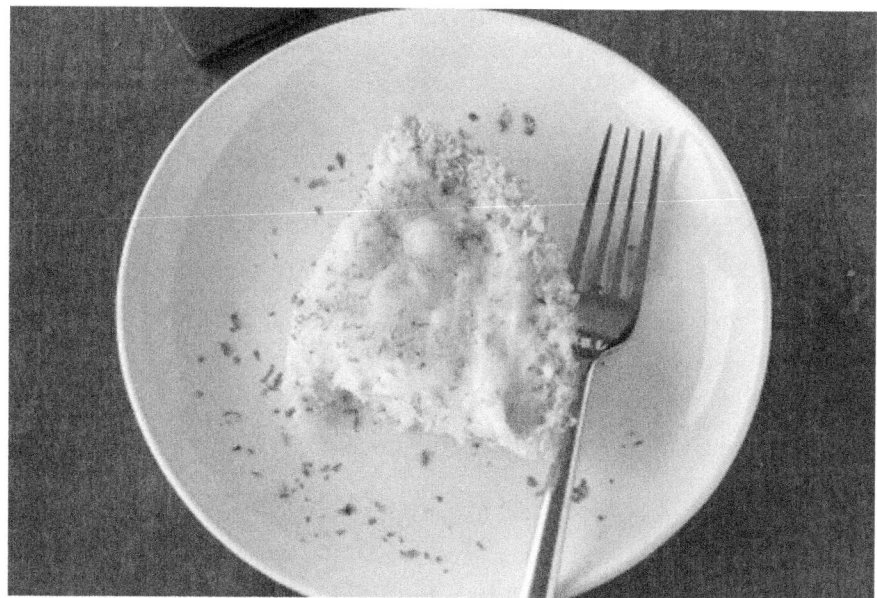

Cooking time: 3 hours   **Servings:** 6

Ingredients:

- 1 head cauliflower, chopped into floret sized pieces
- 2 eggs
- 1 cup cheese blend (cheddar or parmesan shredded cheese blend)
- 1 teaspoon dried Italian seasoning
- ½ teaspoon dried rosemary
- ¼ teaspoon salt
- 4 oz homemade low carb Alfredo sauce

For sauce:

- 1 oz butter, unsalted
- 1 cup heavy cream
- Salt, pepper, taste
- 4 oz parmesan cheese, shredded

Instructions:

1. Put cauliflower florets into a food processor and blend thoroughly.

2. Put blended cauliflower into a bowl, add eggs, seasoning, salt and ¼ cheese. Mix well.

3. Add some oil into a slow cooker or use a cooking spray. Put cauliflower mixture into slow cooker and press down to form pizza base. The edges should be slightly higher around all sides.

4. To cook a low carb Alfredo Creamy Sauce, melt unsalted butter in a medium sauce pan. Add cream and stir well. Add parmesan cheese, 2 tablespoons at a time and stir constantly until incorporated. Add salt and pepper to taste, keep cooking until the sauce thickens.

5. Pour the sauce and the rest of a cheese blend onto the pizza base.

6. Close the slow cooker lid but leave a small space using a woode spoon handle.

7. Cook on High for 2-3 hours. Check if the eggs and crust are cooked well.

8. Let the pizza sit for 20-30 minutes before serving.

Nutritional info:

Calories 105; Fats 5.8g; Net carbs 3.1g; Protein 7.9g

Poached Salmon

Cooking time: 1 hour   **Servings:** 4

Ingredients:

- 4 medium salmon fillets
- 8 oz water
- 2 tablespoons dry white wine
- 1 yellow onion, sliced
- ½ lemon, sliced
- ½ teaspoon salt
- ¼ teaspoon garlic powder
- ¼ teaspoon dried basil

Instructions:

1. Pour water and wine into a slow cooker. Heat on High for 30 minutes with the lid open.
2. Season salmon fillets with salt, garlic powder and basil.
3. Put salmon into slow cooker. Add onion and lemon onto salmon fillets.
4. Close the lid and cook on High for 20-30 minutes.

Nutritional info:

Calories 273; Fats 21g; Net carbs 4.2g; Protein 35g

Cod and Vegetables

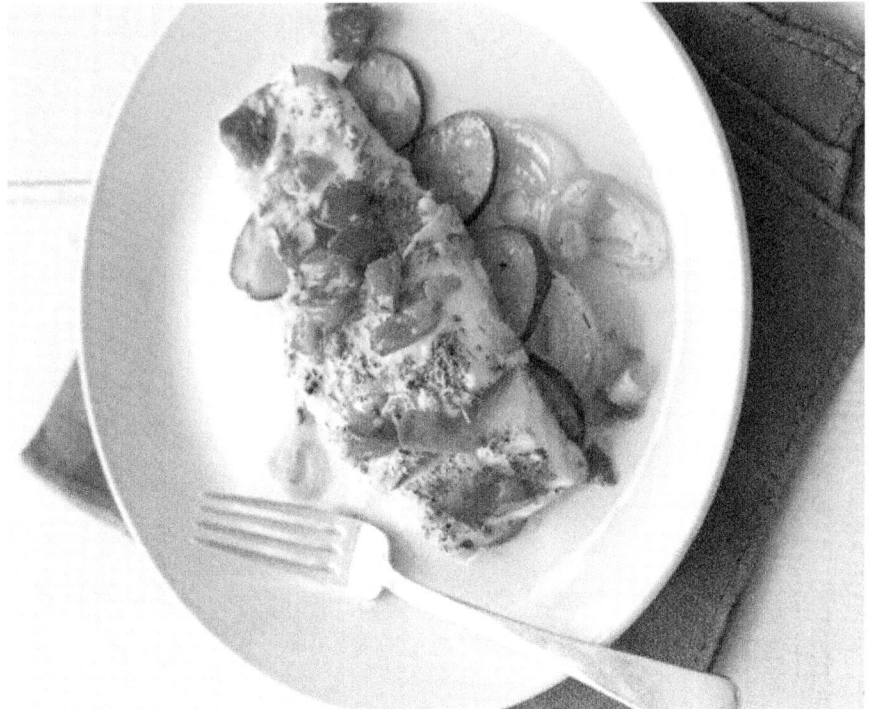

Cooking time: 1-3 hours **Servings:** 4

Ingredients:

- 4 (5-6 oz) cod fillets
- 1 bell pepper, sliced or chopped
- 1 onion, sliced
- ½ fresh lemon, sliced
- 1 zucchini, sliced

- 3 garlic cloves, minced
- ¼ cup low-sodium broth
- 1 teaspoon rosemary
- ¼ teaspoon red pepper flakes
- salt, pepper, to taste

Instructions:

1. Season cod fillets with salt and pepper.
2. Pour broth into slow cooker, add garlic, rosemary, bell pepper, onion and zucchini into slow cooker.

3. Put fish into your crockpot, add lemon slices on top.

4. Close the lid and cook on Low for 2-3 hours or on High for 1 hour.

Nutritional info:

Calories 150; Fats 11.6g; Net carbs 6.2g; Protein 26.9g

Veggie Shrimps

Cooking time: 2-5 hours   **Servings:** 3

Ingredients:

- 1 lb raw shrimps, peeled
- 2 red bell peppers, sliced
- 2 green bell peppers, sliced
- ½ onion, sliced
- 1 small tomato, quartered

- 1 teaspoon salt
- 1 teaspoon chili powder
- ½ teaspoon paprika
- ½ cup low-sodium broth

Instructions:

1. Pour broth into slow cooker. Add bell peppers, tomato, onion, salt and pepper.
2. Close the lid and cook on Low for 5 hours or on High for 2 hours.
3. Season shrimps with paprika and chili powder.
4. Put shrimps into slow cooker, coat well with the broth mixture.
5. Close the lid and cook on High for 30-45 minutes.

Nutritional info:

Calories 111; Fats 21.5g; Net carbs 4.8g; Protein 16.1g

Fish Stock

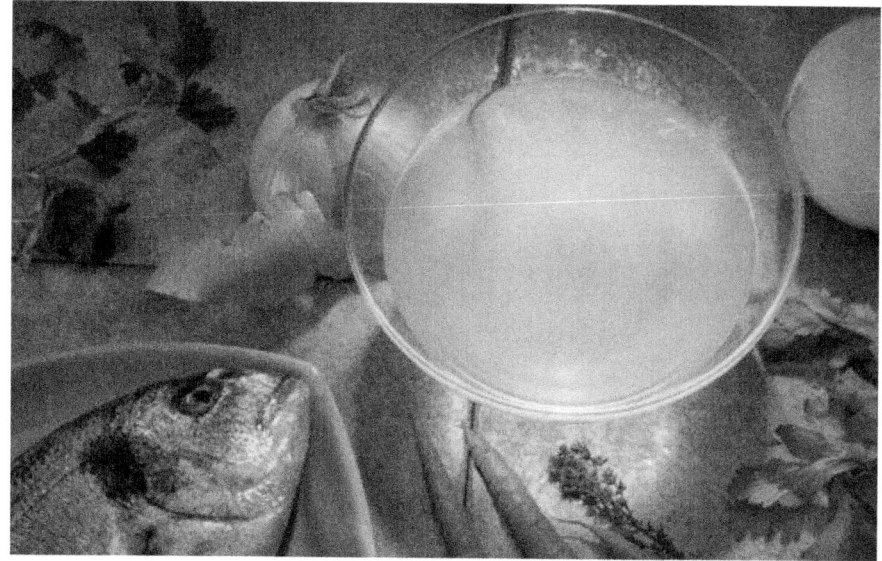

Cooking time: 4-8 hours   **Servings:** 6

Ingredients:

- 2 lb fish heads and bones, gills removed
- 1 tablespoon olive oil
- 1 onion, sliced
- 1 carrot, sliced
- 2 bay leaves
- 1/3 cup parsley stems
- 1/3 cup dill stems
- 2 tablespoons dry white wine
- ½ teaspoon rosemary
- ½ teaspoon dried thyme
- salt, pepper, to taste
- 11 cups water

Instructions:

1. Heat oil in a slow cooker on High. Add onion, cook until translucent stirring constantly.

2. Add carrot, parsley and dill stems, stir for 1 minute. Pour wine into the pan and sauté for 2 minutes.

3. Transfer the vegetables and wine mixture into a slow cooker, add fish. Add salt, pepper, rosemary and dried thyme. Pour water to cover the fish by 1 inch.

4. Close the lid and cook on Low for 6-8 hours or on High for 3-4 hours.

Nutritional info:

Calories 40; Fats 11g; Net carbs 0g; Protein 5.27g

Pollock Stew

Cooking time: 3-5 hours   **Servings:** 6

Ingredients:

- 2 lb Pollock fillets
- 1 onion, chopped
- 3 garlic cloves, minced
- 1 small red chili
- ½ can of 14 oz diced tomatoes, not drained

- ¼ cup parsley, chopped
- 2 tablespoons olive oil
- 1 ½ cup water
- 1 tablespoon dry white wine (optional)
- salt, pepper, to taste

Instructions:

1. Pour oil into slow cooker, add onion, garlic, chili and parsley. Then add tomatoes (with liquid), 1 cup water and wine.

2. Close the lid and cook on Low for 5 hours or on High for 3 hours.

3. An hour before the broth is ready open the lid and add fish, ½ cup water, salt and pepper. You can add some more parsley at this step.

4. Close the lid and cook till the end.

Nutritional info:

Calories 188; Fats 16.1g; Net carbs 3.4g; Protein 19.9g

Trout & Broccoli Chowder

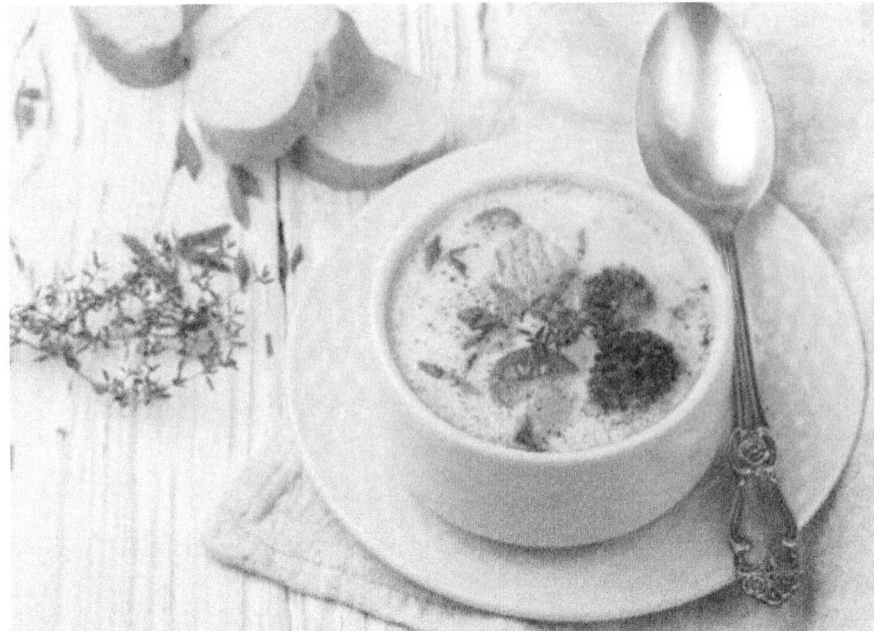

Cooking time: 2 hours   **Servings:** 6

Ingredients:

- 12 oz trout fillets, skin removed
- 1 onion, chopped
- 1 tablespoon butter, unsalted
- 1 cup soy milk, unsweetened
- 1 cup water
- 1 package (10 oz) frozen broccoli, thawed
- ¼ teaspoon garlic powder
- salt, pepper, to taste
- 1 cup cheddar cheese, shredded
- 1 tablespoon parsley, chopped

Instructions:

1. Melt butter in a pan over high heat, add onions. Sauté for 2-3 minutes until onion softens.

2. Transfer onion to a slow cooker. Add milk, broccoli, cheese, fish, garlick powder and salt.

3. Close the lid and cook on High for 2 hours. Check if the fish is soft.

4. Serve topped with parsley.

Nutritional info:

Calories 403; Fats 20.9g; Net carbs 6.7g; Protein 15.2g

Garlic Shrimp

Cooking time: 1 hour   **Servings:** 4

Ingredients:

- 1 lb large or jumbo shrimps, peeled
- 2 tablespoons butter
- ¼ cup olive oil
- ¼ tablespoon cayenne pepper
- 2 teaspoons paprika
- 4 garlic cloves, sliced
- ¼ teaspoon black pepper
- salt, to taste
- 1 tablespoon parsley, chopped
- 1 tablespoon fresh lemon juice

Instructions:

1. Add butter, oil, garlic, paprika, cayenne pepper, salt and black pepper into slow cooker. Close the lid and cook on High for 25 minutes.

2. Add shrimps to the slow cooker and stir well to coat them with oil minture.

3. Close the lid and cook on High for 30 minutes. Stir the shrimps at least once, in 10-15 minutes.

4. Serve topped with parsley and sprinkled with lemon juice.

Nutritional info:

Calories 250; Fats 28.6; Net carbs 2g; Protein 10.8g

Shrimp Creole

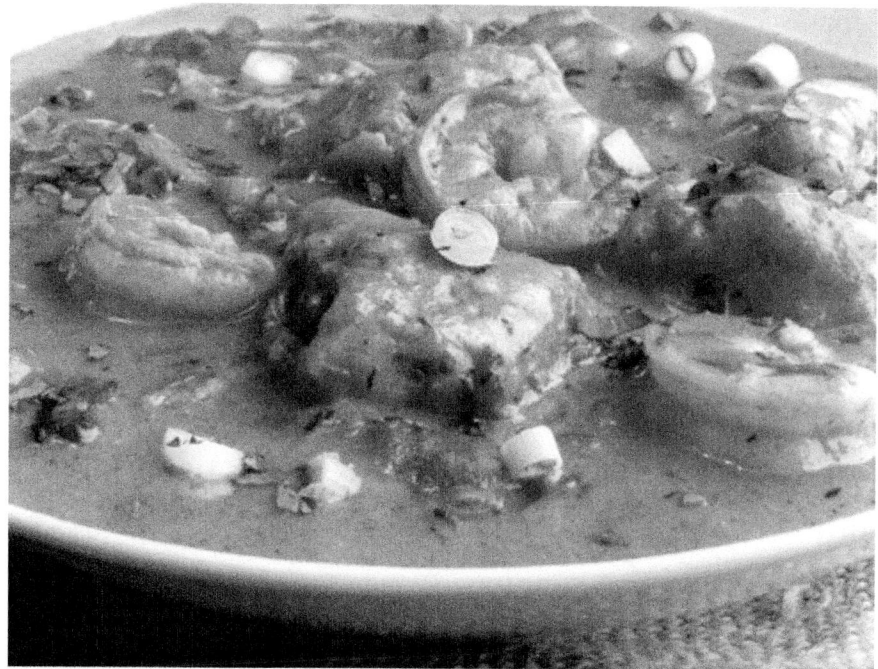

Cooking time: 4-8 hours   **Servings:** 4

Ingredients:

- 1 ½ lb shrimps, deveined
- 1 stalk celery, diced
- 1 onion, chopped
- 1 bell pepper, chopped
- 8 oz tomato sauce
- 1 cup tomatoes, chopped
- 1 garlic clove, minced
- salt, pepper, to taste

Instructions:

1. Add celery, onion, bell pepper, tomato sauce, tomatoes, garlic, salt and pepper to the Crockpot.
2. Close the lid and cook on Low for 6-8 hours or on High for 3-4 hours.
3. Add shrimps to the Crockpot in the last 30 minutes of cooking cycle.

Nutritional info:

Calories 161; Fats 11.8; Net carbs 9.2g; Protein 18.8g

Fish Curry

Cooking time: 2-4 hours   **Servings:** 5

Ingredients:

- 2 pounds cod fillets, cut into medium sized pieces
- 1 onion, diced
- 2 garlic cloves, chopped
- 1 tablespoon fresh ginger, grated
- 1 inch fresh turmeric
- 1 teaspoon coriander seeds
- 1 teaspoon ground cumin
- ¼ teaspoon fenugreek seeds
- 1 tablespoon curry powder
- 2 cups coconut milk
- salt, pepper, to taste

Instructions:

1. Add onion, garlic, ginger, turmeric, coriander, cumin, fenugreek and curry powder to a food processor. Blend until smooth.

2. Pour the mixture into a medium saucepan, add coconut milk and simmer for 5-7 minutes over medium heat.

3. Transfer to the Crockpot, add salt and pepper, close the lid and cook on Low for 4 hours or on High for 2 hours.

4. Season fish fillets with salt and pepper, add to the Crockpot after the sauce has been cooked and cook on Low for 20 more minutes.

Nutritional info:

Calories 446; Fats 35.8; Net carbs 9.8g; Protein 48.9g

Tuna Steaks

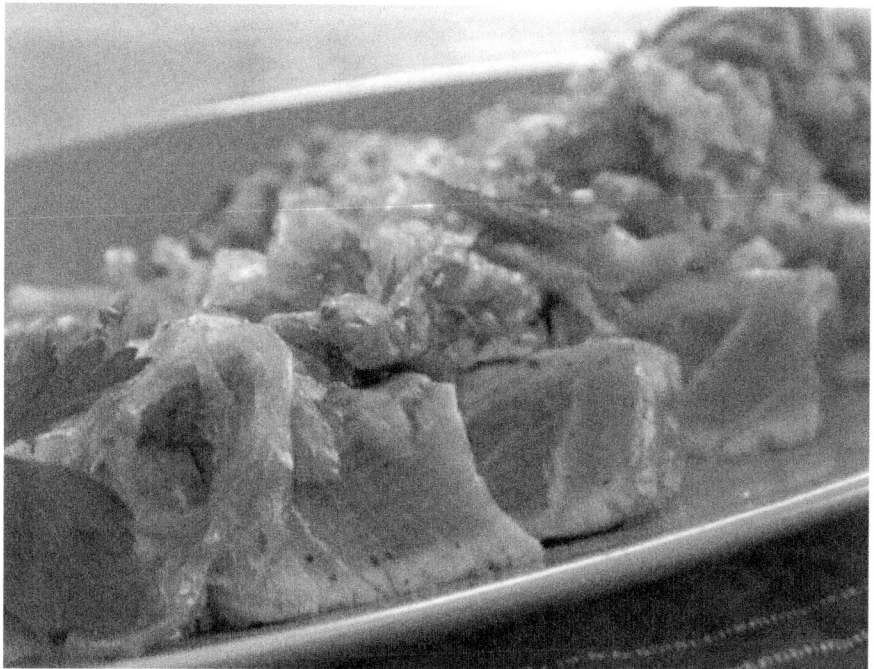

Cooking time: 30 minutes   **Servings:** 4

Ingredients:

- 2 pounds tuna steaks
- 1 onion, sliced
- 1/3 cup white wine
- 5 oz chicken or fish stock
- 1 tablespoon olive oil

- 1 tablespoon lemon zest
- 1 teaspoon ground ginger
- 1 teaspoon coriander
- ½ teaspoon cinnamon
- salt and pepper, to taste

Instructions:

1. Heat oil in a skillet over medium heat. Add onions and cook for 2-3 minutes until soft.

2. Add wine, stock, lemon zest , ground ginger, coriander, cinnamon, salt and pepper. Cook until boils, stirring constantly.

3. Pour the cooked sauce into the slow cooker.

4. Add tuna steaks, close the lid and cook on High for 15-20 hours.

Nutritional info:

Calories 446; Fats 35.8; Net carbs 9.8g; Protein 48.9g

Mixed Seafood Stew

Cooking time: 30 minutes   **Servings:** 6

Ingredients:

- 2 pounds seafood
- ½ onion, sliced
- 2 garlic cloves, minced
- 1 can diced tomatoes
- 4 cups vegetable broth
- ½ cup white wine
- ½ teaspoon thyme
- ½ teaspoon basil
- ½ teaspoon red pepper flakes
- salt and pepper, to taste

Instructions:

1. Pour broth and wine into the slow cooker.
2. Add onion, garlic, tomatoes, thyme, basil, red pepper flakes, salt and pepper.
3. Add seafood, mix well. Close the lid and cook on High for 1 hour.

Nutritional info:

Calories 192; Fats 22.3; Net carbs 8g; Protein 35.3g

Seafood Scampi

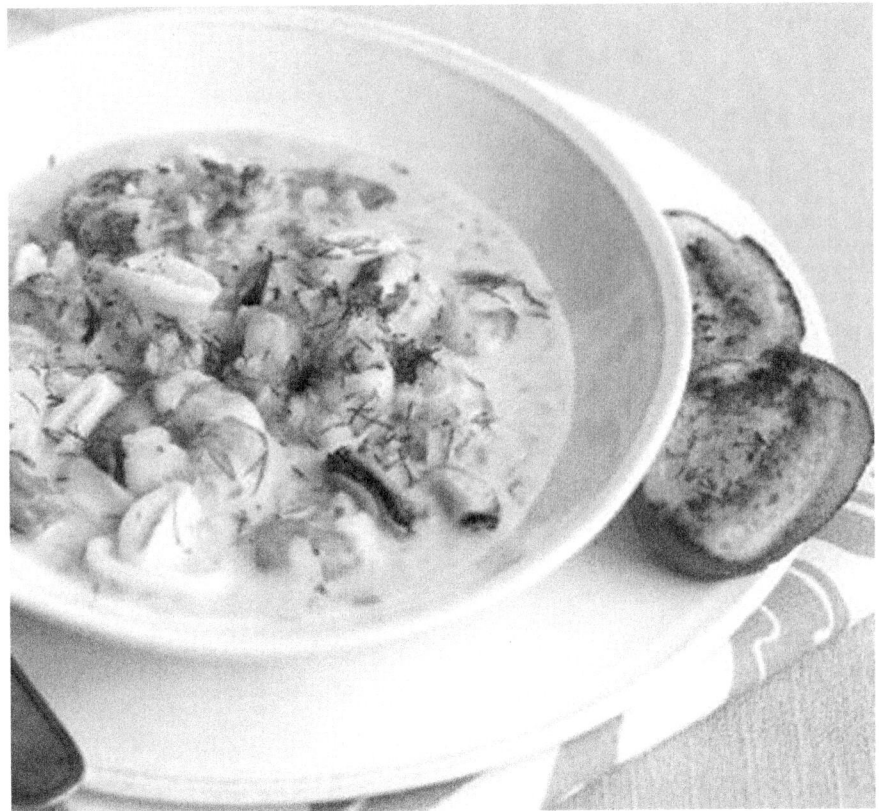

Cooking time: 1-2 hours   **Servings:** 6

Ingredients:

- ½ lb shrimp
- ½ lb scallops
- ½ lb mussels
- 1 cup chicken broth
- 2 tablespoons dry white wine

- 3 tablespoons lemon juice
- 2 tablespoons olive oil
- 4 garlic cloves, minced
- 1 tablespoon parsley, chopped
- salt, pepper, to taste

Instructions:

1. Mix broth, wine, lemon juice, olive oil, garlic and parsley in a slow cooker.

2. Add shrimps, scallops and mussel, add salt and pepper, stir well to coat the seafood.

3. Close the lid and cook on Low for 2 hours or on High for 1 hour.

Nutritional info:

Calories 178; Fats 16.8g; Net carbs 4.4g; Protein 20.5g

Lemon Cake

Cooking time: 3 hours   **Servings:** 6

Ingredients:

- 1 cup coconut flour
- 1 cup almond flour
- 2 eggs
- 2 lemons zests
- ½ cup whipping cream
- ½ cup butter, melted
- 2 tablespoons butter, melted
- 2 teaspoons baking powder
- 5 tablespoons Pyure sweetner
- lemon juice from 2 lemons
- ½ cup boiling water

Instructions:

1. Mix coconut and almond flour, 2 tablespoons sweetener and baking powder in a bowl.
2. Mix eggs, ½ cup butter, whipping cream, lemon juice and lemon zest in a separate big bowl. Whisk well.
3. Add flour mixture to the egg and butter mixture and mix well until combined.
4. Line a slow cooker skillet with parchment paper. Spread the cake mixture into slow cooker.
5. Mix 3 tablespoons sweetener, boiling water, 2 tablespoons butter and 2 tablespoons lemon juice.
6. Add the topping mixture to the slow cooker over the cake base.
7. Close the lid and cook on High for 2-3 hours. Check if the cake is cooked with a toothpick. Insert it in cake center, it should come out clean.

Nutritional info:

Calories 350; Fats 32.6g; Net carbs 10.1g; Protein 17.6g

Low Carb Apple Bread

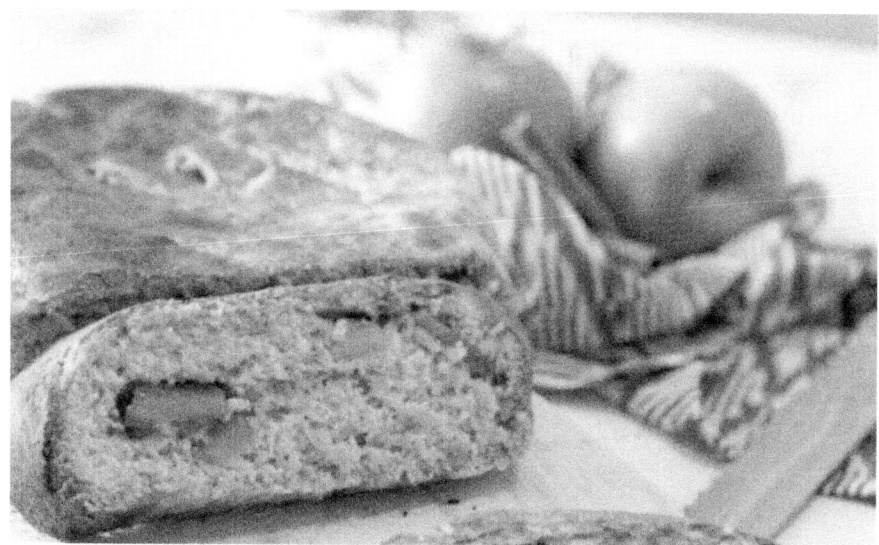

Cooking time: 3 hours   **Servings:** 6

Ingredients:

- 2 cups almond flour
- 1 tablespoon coconut flour
- ¼ cup almonds, chopped
- 1 cup apple, thinly sliced
- 2 eggs
- ¼ teaspoons salt
- 1 teaspoon baking soda
- 3 tablespoons coconut oil
- ½ teaspoon Ceylon cinnamon
- ½ cup Pyure or Swerve sweetener
- 1/3 cup full fat almond or coconut milk
- 1 teaspoon apple cider vinegar
- ¼ teaspoon vanilla extract

Instructions:

1. Mix almond and coconut flour, cinnamon, salt, baking soda and sweetener in a big bowl.
2. Mix coconut or almond milk, coconut oil, eggs, vanilla extract and apple vinegar in a separate medium bowl.
3. Pour milk mixture into the flour mixture and mix well until combined.

4. Add apple and almonds into the bread mixture.

5. Line a slow cooker skillet with parchment paper. Spread the bread mixture into slow cooker.

6. Sprinkle some chopped almonds on top of bread.

7. Close the lid and cook on Low for 2-3 hours. Check if the bread is cooked with a toothpick. Insert it in bread center, it should come out clean.

Nutritional info:

Calories 279; Fats 25.6g; Net carbs 3.6g; Protein 8.1g

Chocolate Chip Zucchini Bread

Cooking time: 3 hours   **Servings:** 6

Ingredients:

- 3 cups almond flour
- 3 eggs
- ½ cup Pyure or Swerve sweetener
- ½ cup vegetable oil
- 1 teaspoon apple cider vinegar
- 1 teaspoon baking soda
- ½ teaspoon baking powder
- 2 teaspoons Ceylon cinnamon
- ¼ teaspoon vanilla extract
- ¼ teaspoon salt
- 1 cup sugar-free chocolate chips
- 16 oz zucchini, peeled, grated

Instructions:

1. Mix eggs, sweetener, vegetable oil and apple cider in a bowl.
2. Mix in flour, baking soda, baking powder, vanilla extract, cinnamon and salt. Mix well until combined.
3. Add zucchini and chocolate chips into the bread mixture.
4. Line a slow cooker skillet with parchment paper. Spread the bread mixture into slow cooker.
5. Close the lid and cook on Low for 2-3 hours. Check if the bread is cooked with a toothpick. Insert it in bread center, it should come out clean.

Nutritional info:

Calories 334; Fats 47g; Net carbs 3.7g; Protein 15.1g

Keto Mocha Fudge Cake

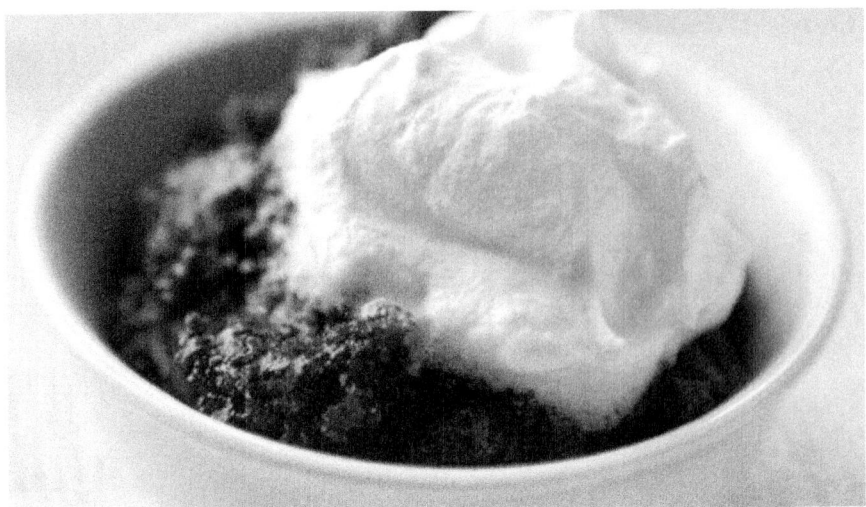

Cooking time: 2-4 hours   **Servings:** 4

Ingredients:

- 2 cups almond flour
- 3 eggs
- 4 tablespoons butter, melted
- ¾ cup sour cream
- ¾ cup hot coffee
- 3 oz unsweetened chocolate, melted

- 1 teaspoon baking soda
- ¼ teaspoon vanilla extract
- ½ teaspoon salt
- 1 ½ cup Pyure or Swerve sweetener

Instructions:

1. Mix butter and sweetener in a medium bowl. Add eggs, chocolate and sour cream, whisk well.
2. Mix in almond flour and baking soda, stir until combined.
3. Add coffee, vanilla extract and salt, mix well.
4. Grease a slow cooker with butter, line it with parchment paper. Spread the cake mixture into slow cooker.

5. Close the lid and cook on Low for 2-4 hours. Check if the cake is cooked with a toothpick. Insert it in cake center, it should come out clean.

6. Serve with whipped cream.

Nutritional info:

Calories 200; Fats 18g; Net carbs 5.8g; Protein 16g

Cranberry Walnut Bars

Cooking time: 2-3 hours   **Servings:** 8

Ingredients:

- 12 oz cranberries, frozen or fresh
- 1 cup water
- 4 ½ oz sweetener
- 1 tablespoon lemon juice
- ¼ teaspoon salt
- ¼ teaspoon nutmeg
- 2 cups almond flour
- 1 cup coconut, finely ground
- ½ cup vanilla whey protein powder
- 8 tablespoons salted butter, melted
- ¾ cup almond meal
- ½ cup walnuts, chopped
- 3 tablespoons brown sugar
- 3 tablespoons sugar-free chocolate chips

Instructions:

1. Mix cranberries, water, 3 oz sweetener, lemon juice, salt and nutmeg in a medium pot and bring to a boil over high heat. Cook for 15 minutes until the cranberry filling thickens. Let it cool.

2. To prepare a shortbread crust, mix almond flour, coconut, protein powder, 1.5 oz sweetener, and pinch of salt in a separate bowl. Pour melted butter onto the flour mixture and mix well until clumps begin to form. Set aside a part of the mixture and save for crumb topping.

3. Line a slow cooker skillet with parchment paper. Put shortbread crust mixture into slow cooker and press down to form bars base.

4. Pour cranberry filling over the base and spread it over it. Sprinkle the walnuts, brown sugar, chocolate chips and reserved shortbread crust over cranberry filling.

5. Close the lid and cook on Low for 2-3 hours. Let cool and cut into 8 bars. Keep refrigerated.

Nutritional info:

Calories 196g; Fats 14g; Net carbs 8g; Protein 10g

Brownies

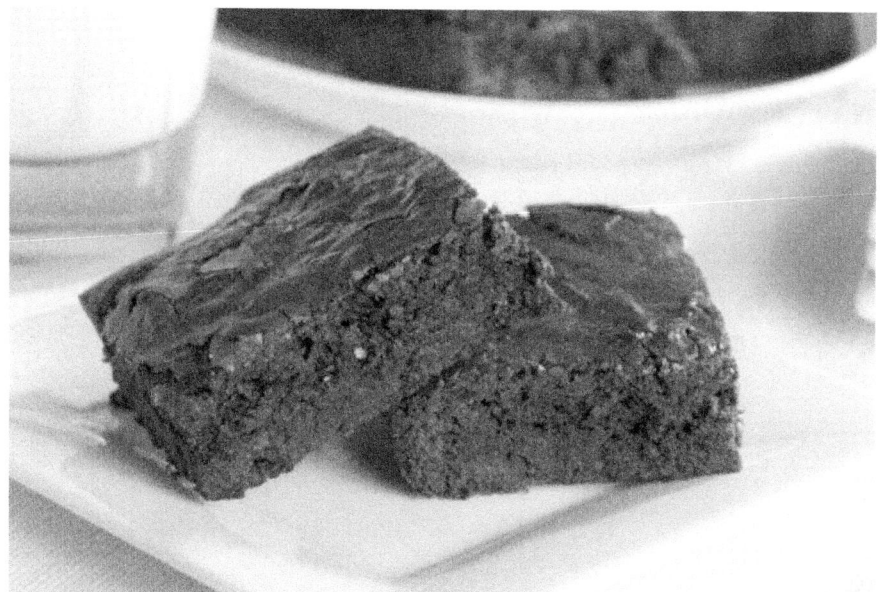

Cooking time: 2-2 ½ hours   **Servings:** 8

Ingredients:

- 4 ½ oz unsalted grass-fed butter
- 1 cup erythritol or brown sugar Truvia
- 2 ½ oz almond flour
- 3 oz cocoa powder
- 2 eggs
- ½ teaspoon salt

Instructions:

1. Mix butter, erythritol, cocoa powder and salt in a saucepan. Heat it over medium heat, stirring constantly. Cook until the sweetener and butter melt.

2. Remove from heat and let the mixture cool a bit.

3. Add one egg at a time, stirring constantly. Add almond flour and mix well until well incorporated.

4. Line your slow cooker with a parchment paper and spray with cooking spray. Pour the batter into the slow cooker.

5. Close the lid and cook on Low for 2-2 ½ hours.

Nutritional info:

Calories 102; Fats 9g; Net carbs 3g; Protein 5g

Pumpkin Pie

Cooking time: 2-3 hours   **Servings:** 8

Ingredients:

- 1 ½ cup almond flour
- 15 oz pumpkin puree
- 2 eggs
- ½ cup unsalted grass-fed butter, melted
- 2/3 cup erythritol or brown sugar Truvia
- ½ teaspoon salt
- ½ teaspoon cinnamon
- ½ teaspoon pumpkin spice

Instructions:

1. Mix butter and erythritol in a bowl.
2. Add eggs one at a time, mix well. Add pumpkin puree.
3. Mix flour, salt, cinnamon and pumpkin spice in a bowl.
4. Add flour mixture to butter and mix well until incorporated.
5. Line your slow cooker with a parchment paper and spray with cooking spray. Pour the batter into the slow cooker.
6. Close the lid and cook on High for 2-3 hours.

Nutritional info:

Calories 102; Fats 9g; Net carbs 3g; Protein 5g

Praline Cheesecake

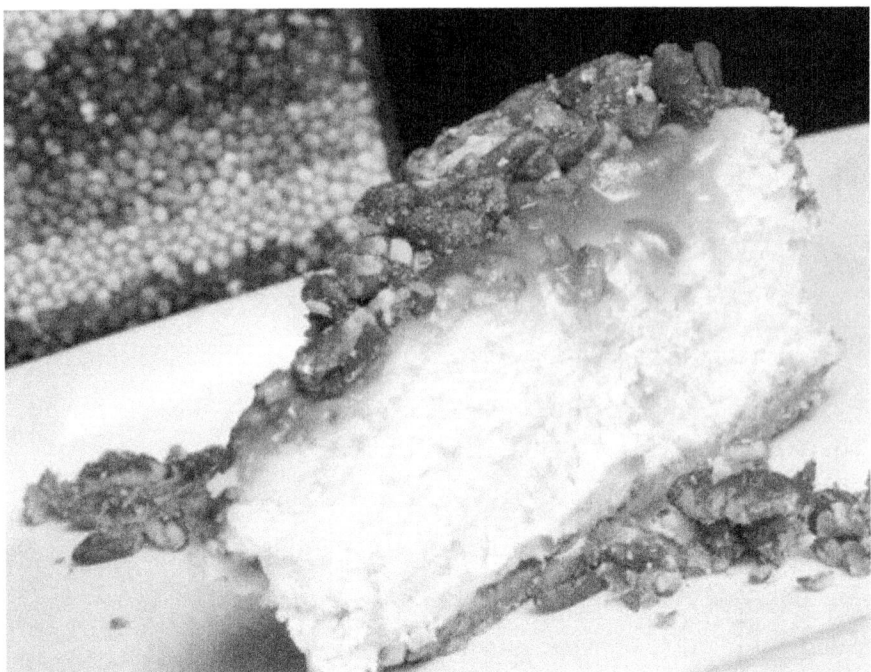

Cooking time: 2 hours   **Servings:** 8

Ingredients:

- 16 ounces cream cheese
- 1 teaspoon butter
- 2/3 cup erythritol or brown sugar Truvia
- 2 eggs

- 1 cup pecans, chopped
- 1 teaspoon pure vanilla extract
- sugar free caramel syrup
- 1 cup water

Instructions:

1. Grease your springform pan with butter. Make sure the pan fits into the slow cooker.

2. Blend cream cheese until creamy and smooth.

3. Add erythritol or brown sugar Truvia and vanilla extract, mix to combine.

4. Add egg, one at a time, keep mixing to combine.

5. Pour caramel on the bottom of the pan, sprinkle with pecans (1/2 cup).

6. Pour cheesecake batter into the pan.

7. Pour water into the cooker, take 3 pieces of foil and make 3 1-inch foil balls. Put the balls into the slow cooker, they will serve as a rack.

8. Put the pan on the foil balls. Close the lid and cook on High for 2 hours.

9. Cover the pan with a foil or a plastic wrap and refrigerate for an hour.

10. Serve garnished with caramel and pecans.

Nutritional info:

Calories 260; Fats 25.3g; Net carbs 2.2g; Protein 16.7g

Ricotta Cheesecake

Cooking time: 2 hours   **Servings:** 8

Ingredients:

- 16 ounces cream cheese
- ½ cup ricotta cheese
- 2/3 cup erythritol or brown sugar Truvia
- ¼ cup sour cream
- 1 tablespoon vanilla extract
- 1 tablespoon lemon juice
- 2 eggs
- 1 cup water

Instructions:

1. Grease a springform pan with a coconut-oil based spray.
2. Mix cream cheese, ricotta cheese, sour cream, erythritol or brown sugar Truvia, vanilla extract and lemon juice, blend until smooth and creamy.
3. Add eggs, one at a time, mix until incorporated.
4. Pour cheesecake batter into your pan.
5. Pour water into the cooker, take 3 pieces of foil and make 3 1-inch foil balls. Put the balls into the slow cooker, they will serve as a rack.
6. Put the pan on the foil balls. Close the lid and cook on High for 2 hours.
7. Cover the pan with a foil or a plastic wrap and refrigerate for 3 hours.

Nutritional info:

Calories 256; Fats 23.6g; Net carbs 6.1g; Protein 7.7g

Berry Sauce

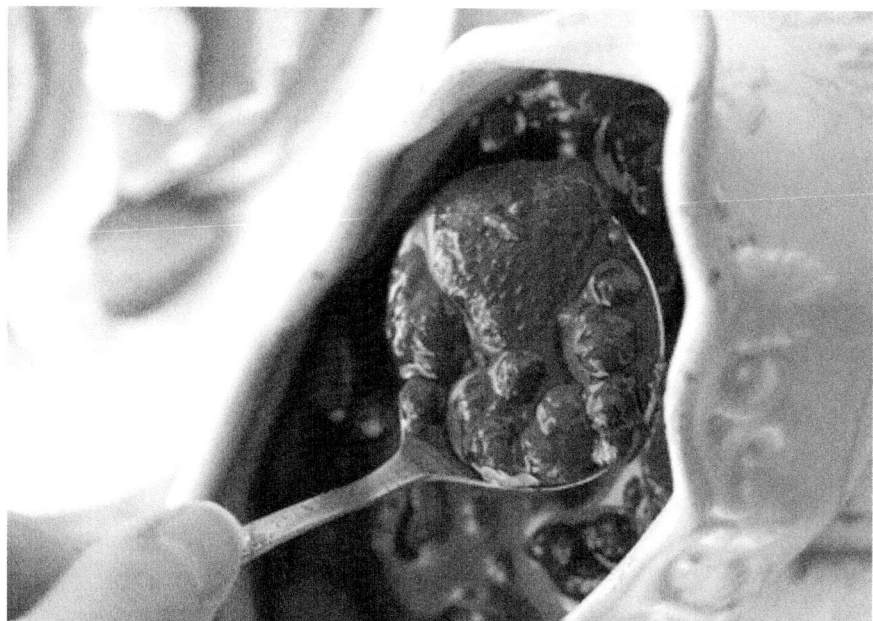

Cooking time: 3 hours   **Servings:** 6

Ingredients:

- 6 oz blackberries, fresh
- 8 oz strawberries, fresh, halved
- 4 oz blueberries, fresh
- ¼ cup Pyure or Swerve sweetener
- ¼ teaspoon xanthan gum (optional)

Instructions:

1. Put blackberries, strawberries, blueberries and sweetener into a slow cooker.

2. Close the lid and cook on Low for 3 hours.

3. 20 minutes before the end of cooking time add xanthan gum if the sauce is not thick enough.

Nutritional info:

Calories 26; Fats 11g; Net carbs 4.7g; Protein 6g

Thank you!

Thank you for purchasing my book! I hope you enjoyed reading and cooking with it. If you can, please leave an honest review for my book, so I and other people know what is good about it or what still needs to be improved. Also, you are more than welcome to check my other book: Ketogenic Instant Pot Cookbook, which is a great addition to this book. https://amzn.to/2Gfcjm8

Thank you one more time!

Printed in Great Britain
by Amazon

42641272R00088